2nd Edition

Connecting with Clients

2nd Edition

Connecting with Clients

Practical Communication for **10** *Common Situations*

DANA DURRANCE, MA
LAUREL LAGONI, MS

AAHA
press

American Animal Hospital Association Press
12575 West Bayaud Avenue
Lakewood, Colorado 80228
800/252-2242 or 303/986-2800
press.AAHAnet.org

Library of Congress Cataloging-in-Publication Data

Durrance, Dana.
    Connecting with clients : practical communication for 10 common situations /
Dana Durrance, Laurel Lagoni. — 2nd ed.
        p. ; cm.
    Laurel Lagoni's name appears first on the earlier ed.
    Includes bibliographical references.
    ISBN 978-1-58326-116-3 (pbk. : alk. paper)
    1. Veterinary medicine. 2. Veterinarian and client. 3. Interpersonal communi-
cation. 4. Pet owners—Psychology. I. Lagoni, Laurel. II. Lagoni, Laurel. Connecting
with clients. III. American Animal Hospital Association. IV. Title.
    [DNLM: 1. Professional-Patient Relations. 2. Veterinary Medicine—methods.
3. Animal Technicians--psychology. 4. Bonding, Human-Pet. 5. Communication.
6. Veterinarians—psychology. SF 745 D948c 2009]
    SF745.L34 2009
    636.089′0696—dc22
                                        2009045418

Printed in the United States of America

10   11   12   /   10   9   8   7   6   5   4   3   2   1

Book design by Erin Johnson Design

I dedicate this second edition to all the amazing veterinary teams who give so much of their heart, expertise, and time toward improving the lives of companion animals. It doesn't matter if you're one of the front staff who checks a patient in, the veterinary technician who inserts a catheter, or the doctor who performs the surgery . . . every single one of you contributes to make veterinary medicine one of the most trusted and respected professions. You are all truly special souls. —D. D.

I dedicate this second edition to the veterinary teams who make emotionally supportive communication a priority in their practices. These professionals know that effective communication doesn't just happen. Rather, it's created by people who take time to learn and then choose to communicate from a place of great respect and empathy. Thank you for establishing a culture of care within your clinical practices and for bringing this sensibility to the field of veterinary medicine. —L. L.

Contents

Acknowledgments

This second edition would not have been possible without the support and expertise of my coauthor, Laurel Lagoni. Twelve years ago, Laurel invited me to write a book with her about communication in veterinary medicine. Over those years, I have enjoyed a wonderful writing partnership with Laurel, not only because she's been a mentor, teacher, and trusted colleague, but also because she's a treasured friend.

For this book to be updated after eleven years, our colleagues at the American Animal Hospital Association Press had to recognize the topic as one that is even more timely and valuable for today's veterinary practice teams. We especially want to thank Bess Maher for her encouragement and guidance during all phases of this project. We would also like to thank Iris Llewellyn and the other editors at AAHA Press for their terrific work.

Equally important are the many talented and hardworking employees at Mountain Shadows Pet Hospital (owned by Dana and her husband, Dr. Steve Durrance) and at World by the Tail, Inc. (owned by Laurel Lagoni and Debby Morehead). All of you bring special qualities to the companies you work for and I'm fortunate to have learned from you. Much of the material in this book was developed and refined based on watching you (from both companies) communicate with and support veterinary clients on an every-day basis.   —D. D.

Writing collaborations are a leap of faith because no two authors approach material in exactly the same way. However, Dana comes as close to the perfect writing partner as I could ever hope for. Exploring and discussing this revision with her has been both enriching and fun. My deepest thanks to you, Dana, for taking on this project with such passion.

Both Dana and I extend our gratitude to the clinicians, veterinary technicians, technicians, residents, interns, students, and other staff members with whom we both worked during our many years of teaching and counseling with the Argus Institute at Colorado State University's James L. Voss Veterinary Teaching Hospital. Drs. Stephen J. Withrow, James L. Voss, Wendell Nelson, and Tony Knight deserve our deepest thanks.

Finally, thanks to W.B. Saunders Company (now Elsevier) and to Carolyn Butler, MS, and Suzanne Hetts, PhD, my coauthors on the groundbreaking textbook *The Human-Animal Bond and Grief* (1994). Although this book is now out of print, many of the concepts included here were developed during the writing of that text.   —L. L.

Preface

All pet owners who truly love their cats, dogs, horses, birds, rabbits, or other animals deserve to have important information conveyed to them with respect, patience, and clarity. It is your responsibility, along with each member of your veterinary team, to ensure this happens.

This book instructs you on *what to say* and *what to do* in a variety of common, though often challenging, client relations situations. The techniques described are most effective when all members of the veterinary team use them consistently.

Every situation offers applied and easily understood information, either to provide quick case references or to serve as a model for veterinary practice team development. In other words, we designed this book to help you and your coworkers get through many of the more difficult and emotional client relations situations you encounter on a day-to-day basis. In these pages, you'll learn how to do the following:

- Increase your knowledge of effective communication and relationship-centered care
- Improve your client relationships and clinical communication skills
- Learn more about shared decision making
- Learn new ways to deal with challenging communication-related situations
- Provide staff training and skill-building exercises
- Increase client retention and loyalty
- Improve staff retention
- Enhance your professional growth and satisfaction with work

Connecting with Clients is intended to guide you toward greater success in the relationships you have with your clients.

How to Use This Book

> " *I hear . . . I forget.*
> *I see . . . I remember.*
> *I do . . . I understand."*
> —Chinese proverb

This book can be used in two primary ways: as a resource and preparatory guide and as a training tool for professional development.

A Resource and Preparatory Guide

There are occasions when you have advance notice before interactions with clients requiring complex and/or skilled communication techniques. In these cases, it is helpful to read about the situation ahead of time and study the material devoted to common communication scenarios. By reading and preparing ahead of time, you will feel more confident about your communication with clients. Your clients may pick up on this confidence and become less anxious and easier to communicate with. Many clients will take their lead from you. If you appear calm, capable, and confident, they in turn will feel calmer in their communication with you.

When reviewing the "10 Common Situations," you will see that all the scenarios described are drawn from everyday situations found in a typical veterinary practice as well as emergency and specialty practices. Recording and occasionally reviewing your notes will help you develop your own unique vocabulary, communication style, and customized reference guide. Write down the phrases, gestures, ideas, and methods your clients seemed to respond to in a positive way so you can be sure to repeat them the next time you're faced with that same situation.

A Training Tool for Professional Development

The Latin word *communis* means "common" and is the root of the word *communication*. When we communicate effectively, we discover the common goals, values, attitudes, and experience we share with others. Common interests allow us to *connect*, or form relationships, finding common ground for problem solving, negotiation, goal setting, and the transference of information.

You might believe some people are just "born communicators," yet experts say effective communication techniques are learned[1] and improve with practice. Olympic swimmers are born with natural talent, but need to work hard to perfect their skills. The comparison holds true for effective communicators.

While the old expression "experience is the best teacher" may be true, it's not always a good thing when you're practicing on real clients in real situations. While real-life experiences are necessary and inevitable, you can also sharpen your skills by using this book as source material for developing role-playing for you and your staff. Role-playing is an incredibly valuable way to train people without the negative outcomes that can occur from practicing on real-life clients.

Role-Playing

Role-playing simply means acting out real-life situations with your colleagues and peers. While it sounds simple and perhaps even artificial, it is the single most effective way to teach, develop, and practice important communication skills. Combined, the authors of this book have over forty years of experience training veterinary professionals. In that time, role-playing has proven to be the single most important teaching tool. That's why, in this book, we've included a sample role-play activity for each common situation discussed, so you can use this book in staff meetings to prepare for situations in which communication can be difficult.

Role-playing usually involves two people (one playing the veterinary professional and the other playing the client). These two individuals then act out specific situations in front of the rest of the staff (who become the audience and observe the action). There are many important benefits to using role-play.

It's the next best thing to real life. You can read and talk about communication skills until the cows come home, but until you actually *use* these skills they are never fully developed. Just as with surgery or any medical procedure, you truly learn by actually *doing* the task and learning from your experiences.

Little risk . . . big gain. Role-playing provides a perfect way to teach and learn difficult material in a fairly safe, nonthreatening environment. If the person playing the role of veterinarian or veterinary professional struggles and messes up, there's no real harm done since real clients in real situations are not involved.

Creative learning means more successful learning. Role-playing provides a unique and even fun way to learn a skill. It challenges you to see not only your perspective in a situation, but the other person's as well. Over the years, many veterinary professionals and students have commented that role-playing makes familiar material seem fresh and different. It allows people to tap into their own creative juices and personal style. This energizes the entire group and as any practice management consultant will tell you, energized groups are more successful groups.

The learning process is often accelerated. People tend to learn and acquire skills more quickly when they are practiced immediately and frequently. This can translate into lower training costs and can free up practice revenue for other things, like employee rewards and raises.

Role-playing promotes group cohesiveness and positive energy. Veterinary teams that regularly role-play rely heavily on experiential learning, which in turn strengthens the dynamics within the team. See the sidebar, "Why Experiential Learning Benefits the Team."

Establishing Ground Rules

The first time role-playing is to be used as a training tool, it is important to set some clear and specific ground rules. Without rules that are fair and enforceable, role-playing can accidentally take a negative turn and actually damage the trust among group members. Therefore, it's best for the facilitator to be a hospital manager or supervisor in the beginning. Once the group becomes familiar with it, other staff members can act as the facilitator. The following guidelines are essential for successful role-playing and should be strictly enforced in a consistent manner.

Make it clear that everyone in the group participates. Whether playing the part as an actor or observing in the audience, everyone has an important

Why Experiential Learning Benefits the Team

Nationally recognized seminar trainer and management coach Micki Holliday believes that there are ten reasons why experiential learning makes groups healthier and more positive.[2]

1. **Clarity**: Role-playing provides and creates more accurate communication by getting into detailed specifics.
2. **Supportiveness**: Role-playing fosters a commitment to stand with, and behind, all group members.
3. **Confidence Building**: Role-playing encourages a personal commitment to improving the self-image of *everyone* in the group.
4. **Mutuality**: Role-playing creates a partnership orientation where the outcome is win-win.
5. **Perspective**: Role-playing allows employees to see things from differing viewpoints (the pet owner, the employee, or even the boss), thereby increasing empathy.
6. **Risk**: Role-playing encourages innovation and places emphasis on the effort made rather than the actual outcome (members are rewarded for taking a risk and being willing to try even if they are not successful).
7. **Patience**: The process of role-playing teaches patience, tolerance, and acceptance of individual communication styles.
8. **Investment**: The more involved group members become in a particular task, the more they will genuinely care about the outcome.
9. **Confidentiality**: Role-playing teaches group members how to protect the information of all team interactions and fosters a sense of trust and comfort with group members.
10. **Respect**: Role-playing forces all group members to give and receive feedback, thus creating mutual respect.

job. While the actors practice new skills, the audience must watch and listen carefully so they can give constructive feedback.

Always ask for volunteers first. For all veterinary teams, the ideal goal is for everyone to take turns at being actors and audience members. Explain that, at first, many of them might feel nervous or shy when they are on stage.

Normalize this discomfort and reassure people that this shyness goes away with time. It is *not* a good idea to force a person to role-play, especially when he or she is vehemently against it! While these reluctant folks are often the ones who would benefit the most from the training, confronting them in this way usually backfires. Allow a person who does not want to role-play when called on to simply say, "I pass." If it becomes obvious that a particular person always passes, you may want to have a private conference to explore ways to encourage him or her.

Use freezing and narrating techniques. This allows participants to freeze the action (like a pause button on a DVD player). When the facilitator needs to interject, he or she can simply say "freeze" and temporarily suspend what's going on. Freezing is also helpful if participants feel stuck or need help from the audience.

To keep role-playing on track, the facilitator might need to comment on the situation unfolding among the actors (by freezing). Through narration, the facilitator can share ideas with the audience about what the actors might be thinking or feeling in a specific situation. For example, "Client X is probably feeling overwhelmed after talking about euthanizing her dog. What do you think would be helpful to do at this point?" Narration may need to be more leading for some situations than for others. If group members are to explore a new skill in a productive way, it is important not to narrate too much. If people are struggling or getting off track, do more narrating.

Set specific guidelines and expectations. Tell the group that it is never okay to hurt anyone's feelings during role-playing even though some role-playing involves acting out a conflict or an argument. Talk with group members about how they can determine if they are hurting someone's feelings (from facial expressions, body language, and so on). Facilitate role-playing in such a way that participants have the flexibility to truly try on new behaviors and issues. This will create an atmosphere of trust, fun, and creativity. It is not helpful, however, to have role-playing that allows so much silliness that the message or the lesson is lost. The facilitator needs to be strong and determined to keep things on track (especially when the audience is giving feedback and can digress to other topics).

One way to "rein in" the role-play is by making sure that people don't act out real-life personal issues. Role-play is *not* the forum for such issues and is inappropriate (after all, this is not group therapy!). Also, it is helpful to remind people not to overact or make the situation difficult for the actors. The idea is to help others learn new skills, not to put them through the ringer. It's okay if participants feel a bit of discomfort (that's how we all stretch ourselves and grow), but it's important not to take it too far.

If you and your coworkers enjoy a fairly high level of trust and mutual respect, it might be interesting to use your experiences with challenging client relationships as the basis of some role-playing. Role-playing allows you to actually try out the words and strategies suggested by others. It also allows you to play the roles of your own clients in order to gain some empathy for their points of view. Participating in role-playing can be intimidating, but if you feel you can trust one another to provide feedback in gentle, constructive ways, try it. Sharing experiences, both rewarding ones and embarrassing ones, is the only way to learn from your own mistakes and successes, as well as those of others. If you are secretive, defensive, and even modest about your own attempts to communicate with and help clients, little progress toward becoming more effective can be made.

Providing Feedback and Debriefing After the Role-Play Has Ended

Research indicates that communication skills are best learned when instructors provide safe, constructive opportunities for practice.[3] In addition to facilitating staff role-play, this goal can be accomplished by providing constructive feedback and debriefing. Feedback that is most helpful contains the following elements:[4]

- **It is solicited, rather than imposed.** Feedback is best when the receiver asks for the information rather than it being imposed by someone else.
- **It is descriptive, rather than evaluative.** When the observer describes only his or her own reactions (descriptive), it prevents the person from feeling defensive and under attack.
- **It is specific, rather than general.** To tell an individual that he or she is dominating is not nearly as useful as saying, "Just now when we were discussing things, you did not listen to what the others said, and I felt a bit forced to accept your arguments."
- **It is helpful to *both* the receiver and the giver.** Feedback can be destructive when it serves our own needs but fails to consider the needs of the person on the receiving end.

- **It is directed toward behavior that the receiver can change.** It is very frustrating when a person is reminded of some shortcomings over which he or she has no control.
- **It is well timed.** Feedback is most useful when it is given shortly after the communication has occurred.
- **It is checked to ensure clear communication**. A way to check this is to have the receivers try to rephrase the feedback they have just received to see if they have an accurate interpretation.

Debriefing

During debriefing, it is important to ask questions that encourage the participants to think and process what's happened. For example, "In this last scenario, what did the veterinarian do that indicated good listening?" Or, "Did the veterinarian do anything that indicated poor listening behavior?"

In general, a debriefing discussion should always begin with open-ended questions. The questions should become more specific as the members' responses become more sophisticated. Let the group's responses drive the questioning. Good questions have the underlying message "I value your ideas and I want to know what you think." This helps maintain an atmosphere in which participants want to volunteer their thoughts, participate in discussions, and push themselves to use higher-order thinking and communication skills. Debriefing is more than venting your frustration. Debriefing means talking openly with your coworkers about your emotional experiences as well as the medical aspects of a case. It also means receiving constructive feedback and support regarding the communication techniques and course of action you chose to take. Here's how you participate in a debriefing session:

- Explain what you felt went well. ("This technique really worked!")
- Explain what you felt didn't go well. ("Mrs. James seemed to get angry with me when I suggested she might want to pay her bill ahead of time.")
- Ask for ideas from your colleagues regarding other ways to handle the situation. ("How do the rest of you deal with suggestions that seem to offend clients?")

Positive interactions between you and your clients lead to deep human connections and relationships. Knowing how to build strong relationships is the heart and soul of any successful business. While positive client relations *will* make your veterinary practice more profitable in the long run—because people will feel more comfortable, understood, and cared about, and thus will return to your practice again and again—client retention and profitability are *not* the main goals of effective communication. The main goals are to truly connect with other human beings and to make each interaction clear, productive, and personally satisfying. A "Role-Play Feedback Form" is provided for you in the Appendix. Feel free to make copies.

Notes

1. P. K. Horvatich and K. B. Meyer, "Teaching Client Relations and Communication Skills: Part III—Preliminary Evaluations of Instructional Effectiveness," *Journal of Veterinary Medical Education,* 7 (1980): 146–150.

2. M. Holliday, *Coaching, Mentoring, and Managing* (Franklin Lakes, NJ: Career Press, 2001).

3. S. M. Kurtz, J. Silverman, and J. Draper, *Teaching and Learning Communication Skills in Medicine* (Abingdon, Oxon, UK: Radcliffe Medical Press, 1998).

4. D. Garland, "Workshop Models for Family Life Education: Couples Communication and Negotiation Skills" (Family Service Association of America, 1978).

Communicating and Connecting

Veterinary Communication

> *What our [medical] system may need is not more intervention, but more conversation . . ."*
> —Ellen Goodman, columnist (*Boston Globe*, May 10, 2009)

Veterinary communication has come a long way since the first publication of this book in 1998. Even a decade ago, communication was considered a "soft science" topic and was taught only occasionally through seminars and conference workshops. Today, several professional veterinary medical schools conduct research in the subject matter and include coursework in clinical communication skills as part of their core curriculum. One veterinary school goes even further and organizes an annual international conference devoted to the topic. In addition, training in health-care communication is sponsored by both corporate and professional veterinary medical groups and offered nationwide, as well as online. At long last, learning to connect or communicate effectively is recognized as critical to the success of veterinary practice![1]

The growing interest in and higher standards for clinical communication are due in large part to the increasing strength and significance of the human-animal bond. Today, over 60 percent[2] of American households include one or more companion animals[3] and, when asked how to characterize their relationships with their pets, 85 percent of pet owners say they view their pets as members of their families.[4] The pet-family bond is a catalyst for change in the way contemporary veterinary medicine is practiced. For example, many clinics now offer bond-centered services (for example, animal behavior counseling, pet loss support, and so on) designed to help *people*, in addition to the high-quality medical care that helps pets.[5]

Bond-centered services are vital to building positive relationships with clients. Experts agree that positive relationships with clients are often the key to success in a practice.[6] It's no wonder, then, that much of the research and teaching currently taking place in the emerging field of veterinary communication is focused on what experts call relationship-centered care.

Relationship-centered care represents a new paradigm in veterinary communication. Characterized by a move away from paternalism and toward partnership, relationship-centered care features shared decision making in order to provide the best care possible for animals.[7] Client-veterinarian partnerships, respect for each family member's perspective, and his or her knowledge of the animal, along with the role the pets play in the family and their financial circumstances, are taken into consideration when recommending treatment plans.

According to studies in human medicine, relationship-centered care is related to more positive health outcomes for patients as well as to the reduction in malpractice complaints.[8] The same may be true in veterinary medicine. A study conducted by the American Animal Hospital Association suggests that most complaints to regulatory bodies are related to poor communication and deficient interpersonal skills, with breakdowns in communication being a major cause of client dissatisfaction. The study also showed a primary reason for noncompliance with a pet's treatment recommendations is inadequate client-veterinarian communication.[9] Many experts believe that practices that prioritize positive client relationships also have higher levels of staff retention, the potential to be more successful financially, and a feeling of being more personally satisfied with work.[10] The benefits of going beyond the medical aspects pertaining to an animal's condition seem clear.

Relationship-centered care includes the exploration and discussion of a patient's lifestyle and biomedical condition as well as building trust and rapport, eliciting a client's concerns, establishing a partnership, expressing empathy, and involving clients in goal setting and decision making.[11] With all that to accomplish, it might seem that the average veterinary team would never have time for a relationship-centered care approach! However, a recent study found that appointments during which only biomedical communication took place were actually, on average, only 1.5 minutes longer than appointments during which the relationship-centered care approach was used.[12] Studies in human medicine have found that the use of appropriate clinical communication skills can improve the accuracy and efficiency of information gathering and adherence to recommendations, resulting in overall time savings.[13,14]

Experts believe there is still a gap between veterinary training and the actual communication skills required to be a successful veterinarian.[15] Several recent studies indicate that, in general, veterinarians lack the knowledge and skills necessary to engage in effective, compassionate communication with clients.[16,17] In one of these surveys, alumni of a veterinary school identified communication skills as one of the topics that should have been addressed during their education.[18]

In human medicine, patients want doctors to be competent professionals *and* sensitive listeners. Surveys in the field of human medicine say patients want their physicians to attend to their emotions and really listen to their concerns.[19] In short, they want to know that their physicians *care*. In fact, studies examining patient satisfaction with human medicine report that *caring* is more valued in the doctor/patient relationship than *curing*.[20] In human medicine, communication is now considered a core clinical skill, along with knowledge, physical examination, and problem solving,[21] with relationship-centered care recognized as a preferred model for doctor-patient interactions. This brief review suggests that veterinary medicine is also moving toward relationship-centered care, and, in accordance with the main message of this book, that's a step in the right direction!

Notes

1. J. P. Brown, "The Current and Future Market for Veterinarians and Veterinary Medical Services in the United States," *Journal of American Veterinary Medical Association* 215 (1999): 161–183.

2. Ibid.

3. American Veterinary Medical Association, *U.S. Pet Ownership and Demographics Sourcebook* (Schaumburg, IL: AVMA, 2007).

4. J. P. Brown, "The Current and Future Market for Veterinarians and Veterinary Medical Services in the United States," *Journal of American Veterinary Medical Association* 215 (1999): 161–183.

5. L. Lagoni, C. Butler, and S. Hetts, *The Human-Animal Bond and Grief* (Philadelphia, PA: W.B. Saunders, 1994).

6. M. A. Stewart, "Effective Physician-Patient Communication and Health Outcomes: A Review," *Canadian Medical Association Journal* 152 (1995): 1423–1433.

7. J. R. Shaw, C. L. Adams, and B. N. Bonnett, "What Can Veterinarians Learn from Studies of Physician-Patient Communication About Veterinarian-Client-Patient Communication?" *Journal of American Veterinary Medical Association* 224, no. 5 (2004): 676–684.

8. Ibid

9. George A. Grieve, Kathleen T. Neuhoff, R. Michael Thomas, Link B. Welborn, John W. Albers, and James C. Parone. *The Path to High-Quality Care: Practical Tips for Improving Compliance* (Lakewood, CO: AAHA Press, 2003).

10. J. R. Shaw, B. N. Bonnett, C. L. Adams, and D. L. Roter, "Veterinarian-Client-Patient Communication Patterns Used During Clinical Appointments in Companion Animal Practice," *Journal of American Veterinary Medical Association* 228, no. 5 (2006): 714–721.

11. J. R. Shaw, B. N. Bonnett, C. L. Adams, and D. L. Roter, *The Path to High-Quality Care: Practical Tips for Improving Compliance* (Lakewood, CO: AAHA Press, 2003).

12. J. R. Shaw, B. N. Bonnett, C. L. Adams, and D. L. Roter, "Veterinarian-Client-Patient Communication Patterns Used During Clinical Appointments in Companion Animal Practice," *Journal of American Veterinary Medical Association* 228, no. 5 (2006): 714–721.

13. M. Stewart, J. B. Brown, W. W. Weston, et al., *Patient-Centered Medicine: Transforming the Clinical Method* (San Francisco: Radcliffe Medical Press, 2003).

14. J. Silverman, S. A. Kurtz, and J. Draper, *Skills for Communicating with Patients* (Abingdon, Oxon, UK: Radcliffe Medical Press, 2005).

15. J. P. Brown, "The Current and Future Market for Veterinarians and Veterinary Medical Services in the United States," *Journal of American Veterinary Medical Association* 215 (1999): 161–183.

16. D. G. Bristol, "Using Alumni Research to Assess a Veterinary Curriculum and Alumni Employment and Reward Pattern," *Journal of Veterinary Medical Education* 29 (2002): 20–27.

17. T. J. Heath, and J. N. Mills, "Criteria Used by Employers to Select New Graduate Employees," *Australian Veterinary Journal* 78 (2000): 312–316.

18. D. G. Bristol, "Using Alumni Research to Assess a Veterinary Curriculum and Alumni Employment and Reward Pattern," *Journal of Veterinary Medical Education* 29 (2002): 20–27.

19. J. Antelyes, "Client Hopes, Client Expectations," *Journal of American Veterinary Medical Association* 197, no. 12 (1990): 1596–1597.

20. R. Peters, *Practical Intelligence* (New York: Harper and Row, 1987), 96.

21. S. M. Kurtz, T. Laidlaw, G. Makoul, et al., "Medical Education Initiatives in Communication Skills," *Cancer Prevention and Control* 3 (1999): 37–45.

Communication Protocols and Clinical Communication Skills

> " *[Animals] are not . . . underlings; they are other nations, caught with ourselves in the net of life."*
> —Henry Beston

Just as there are many kinds of veterinary medical care—like routine, palliative, and emergency—there are also many types of clinical communication. For example, the interview skills required to elicit information from a client during a wellness appointment may be quite different from those needed to facilitate a problem appointment or to comfort a client whose pet has just died.

When cases involve special circumstances or human emotions, they require a communication plan that aims toward building caring client relationships as well as conveying medical information. A communication plan or protocol provides direction as well as training material for your entire practice team. Written and well-rehearsed protocols help you and your staff understand *who* is responsible for each step of the communication process as well as *when* each step should be implemented.

Practice teams committed to skilled communication use protocols, along with specific communication skills, to deal with common yet challenging situations like medical emergencies, patient death, and angry clients more efficiently and effectively. You wouldn't begin surgery without knowledge of anatomy and the proper instruments and equipment. Likewise, you shouldn't begin the communication process without appropriate communication techniques. Creating a specific plan and using clinical communication skills for emotionally challenging client interactions is no less important than the protocols and appropriate tools for medical treatment.

Communication Protocols

Every communication process is made up of four basic elements.[1] Here are the first three:

1. The sender: the person who speaks or conveys the message that is intended to be sent.
2. The message: usually an idea, thought, emotion, or piece of information.
3. The receiver: the listener or observer, the person for whom the message is intended.

When these three elements work effectively, they create a feedback loop. In a feedback loop, the roles of sender and receiver alternate and information is passed back and forth successfully.

However, sometimes the message that is received is not the one you intended to send. Receivers determine the meaning and significance of the words you speak based on many other considerations, such as the gestures you use, your facial expressions, and even your tone of voice. Messages are also influenced by time, the environment, and the nature of the relationship between you and the person with whom you are communicating. Thus, here is the fourth element of communication:

4. The interpretation:[2]

If clients misinterpret your comments or behaviors and believe you are judging or trivializing the deep feelings they have for their pets, the trust or relationship that exists between you may become damaged. Likewise, when client relations issues like complaints, anger, or grief are not acknowledged with sincerity and respect, clients may become dissatisfied, disillusioned, and even hostile. You can avoid upsetting encounters like these by creating communication plans that assist you in building positive relationships with clients.

The following outline has been used in well-established clinical teaching programs[3] and can be used to design communication protocols for your practice. Before adapting your own protocols to this outline, identify the type of interaction required and the goal or outcome you want to achieve.

STEP 1 Lay the Foundation

- Create a physical environment conducive to clear, comfortable communication and for providing emotional support, if needed (for example, comfort rooms, private consultation and telephone areas, a private bench in a quiet corner, or a blanket laid on the grass in an outdoor setting).
- Stock supplies and equipment that assist team members in their efforts to provide relationship-centered care (to build trust and rapport, provide emotional support, and so on). These items might include tissues, client handouts, educational videos, beverages, consent forms, or prepackaged paw print kits.
- If necessary and appropriate, establish a written fee structure for any nonmedical appointments or consultations that may be necessary to deal with your clients' needs, such as pet loss counseling provided through your practice.
- Anticipate your clients' needs for convenience, comfort, and access to staff (provide comfortable chairs in the waiting area, be available at a certain time of the day via e-mail, and so on).
- Assign specific support roles and tasks to staff members.

STEP 2 Conduct the Communication

- Establish trust and rapport (discuss the policies and values of your practice, acknowledge the special bond between the client and pet, validate the client's emotions).
- Use appropriate clinical communication skills to educate, create client-veterinarian partnerships, share decision making, meet your clients' emotional needs, and/or facilitate the resolution of a conflict or misunderstanding.
- Adapt your medical procedures so they can easily be understood and observed by your clients, if possible.
- Provide your clients with value-added products to nurture the relationship between them and the practice (children's books about responsible pet care, animal behavior management toys, ClayPaws® prints as keepsakes following euthanasia, or animal neck scarves after routine examinations or vaccinations).

STEP 3 Stay Connected Through Follow-Up Care

- Connect with your clients by e-mail, telephone, or scheduled appointments to evaluate the status of their pet, as well as their own satisfaction with your care.
- Update your records.
- Send a written communication, if appropriate (a condolence card with grief education enclosures, referral recommendations and information, or thank-you notes).
- Debrief the case with the staff members who were involved, if necessary.
- Review and/or role-play the case during your weekly staff meeting so you can all learn more about which techniques worked well and which ones weren't as effective. Break each communication down into specific skills and discuss whether or not the verbal communication matched the nonverbal. Did an inconsistency cause confusion?

Also refer to the "Three-Step Emotional Support Protocol Planning Form" in the Appendix as you the establish your practice's communication protocols.

Clinical Communication Skills

The general consensus is that clinical communication skills and relationship-building techniques can be taught—and learned![4] The following skills are proven essentials for building relationships and can be used to implement your communication protocols. Before using these skills, identify the outcome you want to achieve and the skills that are most likely to help you meet your goals. Keep in mind that several skills can be used simultaneously.

Nonverbal Communication

You may be surprised to learn that the majority of messages sent between people are conveyed nonverbally. In fact, psychologist Albert Mehrabian says that only 7 percent of our ideas and emotions are communicated to one another with words.[5] More specifically, Mehrabian has found that 38 percent of a message's impact comes from vocal cues (voice tone, volume, pitch, rhythm, and so on) and 55 percent from body movements (facial expressions, hand gestures, and posture). That means that 93 percent of our thoughts, ideas, and feelings are communicated without words.

Nonverbal communication is also *what* is said, *where* it is said, *how* it is said, *why* it is said, *when* it is said, and to *whom* it is said. It is also what is *not* said. The nonverbal part of communication is important because it helps people interpret or add meaning to what they are hearing. For example, as you work with clients, begin to notice how their body language and eye contact differ from one situation to another. Start by observing how unhappy or angry clients use closed body language and divert their eyes while happy or confident clients use open body language and direct eye contact. Notice also how your clients' use of direct and indirect eye contact and open or closed body posture evokes the same responses from you. Remember, in a communication feedback loop you alternate between the positions of sender and receiver. Therefore, watch your clients' eye contact and body language—and be aware of your own as well!

When we communicate, we expect that people's words will match their facial expressions, gestures, tone of voice, and body language. If their words say one thing and their actions say something else, it can be very confusing. Therefore, nonverbal and verbal communication must be congruent.

The term *congruence* means "agreement of fit."[6] It means that your nonverbal and verbal messages are compatible and that the message given verbally matches the one that is broadcast by your body.

Nonverbal Communication Skills

Structuring the Environment

When emotions are high, people tend to get frozen into position. They forget they can stand up if they're sitting, walk around the room if they're standing, or even leave the room altogether if they need a few minutes to be alone. This rigidity can be overcome by adapting the physical elements of your environment to better meet whatever situation is at hand.

Structuring the environment means paying attention to the various elements of your office, examination rooms, and consultation areas that can easily be moved and changed, including how chairs are arranged and how the furnishings in the room convey comfort, warmth, and understanding. The goal of structuring the environment is to invite your clients to communicate about their emotions instead of covering them up.

Structuring the environment might mean grouping chairs so conversations can take place face-to-face without barriers like desks or examination tables between you and your clients. It could also mean adapting examination rooms so euthanasia can be performed on the examination table, the floor, or even on a gurney rolled over near the window so the pet and pet owner can be near the outdoors together.

Attending

Attending makes use of body language to convey that careful attention is being paid to the person who is talking. When your body posture is open, your eye contact is direct, and you are leaning slightly forward toward the speaker, you are demonstrating your availability and willingness to be of service.

Attending behaviors include nonjudgmental facial expressions, encouraging gestures, affirmative head nods, and direct observation of what is occurring. Examples of attending behaviors include sitting down if your client sits down and squatting down to be at a child's eye level when greeting or talking to him or her directly.

Active Listening

There is a difference between *merely hearing* your clients and *actively listening* to what they say. Active listening means listening for feelings rather than just the factual content of conversations. Active listening incorporates paraphrasing, asking questions, and attending behaviors such as eye contact and open body posture in order to encourage clients to say more. Two minor, but nevertheless important, nonverbal active listening techniques are necessary silences and minimal encouragers:

1. **Necessary silences.** When emotions are high, it is tempting to babble in order to fill the silence in a conversation; yet remaining silent while others gather their thoughts or vent their feelings is often far more helpful.

2. **Minimal encouragers.** Minimal encouragers are simple responses that encourage people to continue talking. The purpose of minimal encouragers is to let people know you are actively participating in the communication taking place between you. Minimal encouragers include head nods, eye blinks, and phrases like "Uh-huh," "I see," and "For instance?"

Responding with Touch

Touch provides comfort, demonstrates care and concern, and often takes the place of reassuring words. Touch often has a calming effect and can help people slow their thoughts and steady themselves emotionally. There is some scientific evidence that touch affects the body physiologically, slowing heart rate and lowering blood pressure. Touch can be used to soothe a grieving client or to bring someone who is rambling back to the point.

When using touch with clients, neutral or safe areas to touch are the shoulders and arms. Areas of the body that are not viewed as neutral or safe include the neck, hands, torso, lower back, and legs. In general, people dislike being patted on their backs or heads. This behavior suggests a sense of superiority on your part and can be viewed as condescending. If touching or hugging clients makes you uncomfortable, a substitute technique is to touch your clients' companion animals carefully. Pet owners often judge your sensitivity based on how you handle their pets.

Demonstrations

Demonstrations are a way to simplify and to walk clients through complicated and overwhelming medical information or procedures. Verbal descriptions generally accompany demonstrations. When used together, verbal descriptions and demonstrations give clients a step-by-step idea about what needs to be done for their companion animals.

When clients have a visual understanding of what certain treatments entail, it is often easier for them to decide whether or not those options are right for them. Videotapes are available that demonstrate the key points of several treatment protocols and surgical procedures. Offering these videotaped demonstrations to your clients to watch, either at your clinic or at home, can also aid their decision-making process.

Written Information

Providing clients with written information is another form of nonverbal communication. Much of the medical jargon and information familiar to you is very foreign-sounding and unfamiliar to average pet owners. Therefore, it helps to write things down or to draw pictures for clients. Drawings and written materials also allow pet owners to take information home so they can describe their pets' situations accurately and in full detail to the other members of their families.

Verbal Communication

With verbal communication, *what* you say is not as important as *how* you say it. The context in which your words are spoken has the greatest impact on the message you are trying to convey.

The effectiveness of verbal communication is affected by the words you choose, your grammar, and the tone, volume, and pitch of your voice. Effectiveness is also affected by the emphasis and inflection you place on certain words and the pacing of your overall speech. Research says that tone and pacing have the most influence on the meaning of spoken words.[7] For instance, if you use appropriate words to describe a situation but speak very fast, you may be seen as rushed, nervous, insensitive, or unsure of yourself. If you speak the same words too slowly, though, you may be viewed as dull, boring, or even condescending. It's especially important for you to control your tone and pacing when you are working with clients who are anxious, angry, grieving, or upset, because words that are spoken softly and at a slightly slower pace than normal are viewed as more soothing and comforting.

The words you use are also important. When health-care professionals use medical jargon, some clients view them as more credible and their confidence in them increases. However, jargon can alienate other clients.[8] Therefore, if technical medical terms must be used, you should also explain them in plain language. For example, the word *lymphoma* is an unknown term to the average pet owner. The word *cancer*, however, is very familiar. Therefore, when delivering the diagnosis of lymphoma, you should also use the word *cancer*. When you and your clients share an understanding of the meaning of words, you connect on common ground. That's when true communication begins.

Verbal Communication Skills

Acknowledging

To acknowledge is to recognize the existence or truth of something. Acknowledging encourages people to deal openly and honestly with both the emotions that arise within them and the reality of the situation at hand. "I understand you're upset because you believe I charged you too much for Dusty's dental exam."

Normalizing

To normalize is to lend credibility to others' thoughts, feelings, and behaviors. This validates their experiences. For example, the symptoms of grief can seem quite disturbing when they are not clearly understood. It is helpful to normalize grief with statements like "I would expect you to cry about Ruby. You two were best friends for ten years. It's normal to miss her."

Giving Permission

Giving permission means encouraging clients to think, feel, and behave however they need to (within safe limits) without fear of judgment. This technique also allows clients to ask for what they want or to make requests that are important to them. For instance, a client who is anxious before his or her pet has surgery may want to wait at your clinic until the surgery is completed. "I know you and Ruby are very close. If you would like to wait here until her surgery is completed, it's perfectly fine with me."

Asking Appropriate Questions

By asking questions, you gain valuable information about the circumstances surrounding your clients' needs, problems, complaints, or concerns. Failure to ask questions can lead to more difficulties, as there are consequences to making assumptions about your clients' needs.

The most helpful questions are open ended, not closed. A closed-ended question can be responded to with "yes," "no," "fine," or another one- or two-word answer. Open-ended questions elicit more detailed information and create opportunities for clients to tell you more about what they are experiencing.

Open-ended questions begin with "how" or "what" rather than with "why." "How" and "what" questions elicit thoughtful explanations. "How can I help you explain Ruby's illness to your daughter?"

"Why" questions often elicit "I don't know" answers. "Why" questions also have a tendency to put clients on the defensive, making them feel they need to explain themselves to you. One word of caution: A well-placed, open-ended question can launch a lengthy client monologue, so don't use it when you have a limited amount of time to spend with clients.

Paraphrasing

Paraphrasing is the restatement or summary of clients' communication in order to test your understanding of their comments. When you paraphrase clients' comments, it reassures them that the intended message got through. It also provides them with the opportunity to clarify what was meant if your understanding is inaccurate.

When paraphrasing words and emotions, it is important to paraphrase voice tone and pacing as well. If a client is speaking quickly and loudly, you should respond in a voice that corresponds in volume and energy. For example, if you paraphrase anger using a slow-paced, quiet voice that is devoid of emotion, your client may feel you are being patronizing. This is likely to elicit more anger or even sarcasm from your client. While you don't want to yell or scream at a client when paraphrasing anger, you do want to speak boldly, using a firm voice. As rapport develops and you gain some control over the situation, lowering your voice and slowing your pace may in turn slow down your client's side of the conversation and create an atmosphere more conducive to communication.

There are many ways to paraphrase. Easy ways to begin paraphrase statements are "It seems like . . . ," "It sounds like . . . ," and "If I hear you correctly, you feel . . ." A final way to use paraphrasing is to summarize the main points of a lengthy conversation in order to ensure that you've understood all of your client's concerns. Here is an example:

> **Client:** "I don't know how I'll ever find the money to treat Ruby's illness."
> **Veterinarian:** "You're worried that you can't afford to help Ruby get better."

Self-Disclosure

Self-disclosure is *briefly* sharing a personal experience when it may be appropriate and of use to clients. Self-disclosure about your own experiences can help your clients feel more connected to you. When using self-disclosure, it is very important not to shift the focus away from your client and onto yourself. An example of effective self-disclosure is "I was unhappy with something my own physician did last month and felt I needed to discuss it with him, yet, like you, I was unsure about how to bring it up in our conversation. I didn't want to offend him or damage our relationship."

Gentle Confrontation

Gentle confrontation can be used to point out discrepancies or inconsistencies in what has been said or done. It can also be used to set limits on clients' behaviors or expectations. Gentle confrontation may take the form of a question or a statement. Here are some examples of gentle confrontation:

> **Client:** "You don't care at all about what happens to me or my dog!"
>
> **Veterinarian:** "I wonder if you really believe that. You've been bringing Ruby to me for almost four years, and together we've helped her through many medical problems. I wonder if your harsh words today are really your anxiety about Ruby's current illness."

> **Client:** "I know it isn't your fault that you were out of town yesterday when I needed you."
>
> **Veterinarian:** "I hear a lot of anger in your voice, and yet you say you're not angry."

Clients in need, or those who are upset or angry, are often demanding and obnoxious. Due to their strong emotions, they may behave in ways that they would otherwise not dream of. Gentle confrontation is a necessary communication technique that will help you set limits. With it, you can sensitively but firmly help clients understand your own limitations as well as the established policies of your practice. For example, you can say something like "It's obvious to me that you are disappointed that you can't stay with Ruby overnight. I know this is upsetting to you. However, I feel I have been very clear with you regarding our policies from the start. As I've said, we do not allow owners to spend the night in our clinic."

Gentle confrontation may also be used to narrow the content of the client's conversation. Some clients ramble on about topics unrelated to animal care, making it difficult for you to cover pertinent topics with them. Clients sometimes steer conversations off track because they don't want to make difficult decisions or hear what you have to say. Gentle confrontation allows you to redirect the conversation. You can say something like "I'd like to hear more about your son's wedding when we have more time, but right now we need to make some decisions about Ruby's treatment before I have to move on to my next patient."

Immediacy

Immediacy combines gentle confrontation and self-disclosure. The purpose of immediacy is to comment on the unspoken feelings or thoughts that exist within an interpersonal relationship. The use of immediacy requires you to talk openly with your clients about what you are feeling or experiencing *right now*. It is an extremely important skill for almost any difficult situation because it allows you to be honest with the other person about your feelings. For example, you might say, "I feel like something just changed between us. Did my last comment offend or hurt you in some way?" Or, "You're telling me that nothing is wrong, yet you seem quite angry and your tone of voice sounds abrupt. Is there something that we need to talk about? I would like us to be honest with each other."

Using immediacy to comment directly on clients' thoughts, emotions, and behaviors may be intimidating, so it is most effective when used within a well-established relationship. If it is used too soon or in a harsh way, clients may feel exposed or judged and react defensively.

A Note About E-mail and Telephone Conversations

The techniques described in this book are intended to be used during face-to-face interaction. We understand that e-mail and telephone conversations can also be powerful communication tools when used by skilled communicators. However, they can also lead to misunderstandings, because the visual cues relied on for the accurate interpretation of words are missing. When using e-mail, text messaging, the telephone, or any other social medium, keep the following points in mind:

- When using the telephone, remember that your voice is your most powerful tool. Pay special attention to your tone of voice, pitch, and the pacing of your words. In addition, prepare yourself for potentially emotional calls by finding a quiet, controlled environment where you won't be distracted or interrupted.

- Do not convey details about emotional topics like a pet's death, relapse, or body care arrangements via e-mail, text message, or voice mail. Instead, ask your client to call you or visit you at your clinic.

- Maintain your client's confidentiality. If another family member or a coworker answers the telephone or returns your call, it may be best to refrain from providing the details of your patient's condition. Simply instruct the person who answers to ask your client to return your call.

- If a client has not returned your e-mail, text message, or call within a reasonable amount of time, contact him or her again. Messages get lost and clients, especially emotional ones, sometimes forget to respond. It's your responsibility to make contact with your client and it's important that you keep trying until that task is accomplished.

- When you contact a client during work hours, he or she may be unable to speak with you about emotional issues, because of a lack of permission and/or the privacy needed to do so. If you do reach your client, explain that you need to discuss a difficult issue before you begin and ask if this is a convenient time to talk. The client might prefer to arrange a telephone appointment instead, when he or she can speak more freely from a private area.

- Give clients choices regarding how much detail and the kind of information you share with them before you include it all in an e-mail or telephone conversation. For example, you might say, "I would be happy to explain the details of Misty's surgery to you. Would you like that information now?" Each client's need for details varies, so it's best to ask rather than overwhelm your clients with information.

Limits of Client Communications

When you recognize the significance of the human-animal bond and become skilled at communication, you often develop a caring (and extremely loyal) clientele. Many of your clients will grow to think of you as a friend. Once they have experienced the quality of your care, they may naturally turn to you for assistance with other problems in their lives. They may come to you with questions about a personal illness they are coping with, their child's struggle to recover from a severe injury, or the death of one of their close relatives or friends. It will be tempting for you to try to help them in some way. Please be cautious, as you can quickly get in over your head if you ignore the limits and boundaries of your knowledge and skills.

Remember to focus your communication on the issues that arise *specific to the treatment of a companion animal*. As much as you'd like to help a client face personal issues, like the impending death of her elderly father, *you are not trained to do so*. Your job is to acknowledge her feelings, express the compassion you feel for her situation, and refer her to an appropriate human service professional. As a veterinarian, your communications with clients should focus only on the thoughts, feelings, behaviors, and problems associated with their companion animals.

A final point to keep in mind is that, while the clinical communication skills and protocols described are designed to be effective with the majority of veterinary clients, individual differences must be considered. For example, your client's age, gender, culture, religious orientation, and other factors can influence how he or she communicates, especially during emotional interactions. Therefore, it's important to remember that beginning your interactions with clients with a realistic assessment of their human/emotional needs and abilities is as important to the effectiveness of your communication as making an accurate diagnosis of your patients' physical condition is to your medical treatment plan.

Notes

1. W. Schramm, ed., "How Communication Works," in *The Process and Effects of Mass Communication* (Urbana: University of Illinois Press, 1954), 3–4.

2. D. K. Berlo, *The Process of Communication: An Introduction to Theory and Practice* (New York: Holt, 1960).

3. D. Morehead, J. Brannan, L. Lagoni, C. Butler, and K. Wheeler, *Guidelines for Bond-Centered Practice* (Fort Collins, CO: Argus Institute, 2001).

4. P. K. Horvatich, and K. B. Meyer, "Teaching Client Relations and Communication Skills: Part III—Preliminary Evaluations of Instructional Effectiveness," *Journal of Veterinary Medical Education* 7 (1980): 146–150.

5. A. Mehrabian, "Communication Without Words," *Psychology Today*, September 1968, 53.

6. D. Thompson, ed., *The Pocket Oxford Dictionary of Current English*, 8th ed. (Oxford: Clarendon Press, 1992).

7. A. Mehrabian, "Communication Without Words," *Psychology Today*, September 1968, 53.

8. J. B. Coe, C. L. Adams, and B. N. Bonnett, "A Focus Group Study of Veterinarians and Pet Owners' Perceptions of Veterinarian-Client Communication in Companion Animal Practice," *Journal of American Veterinary Medical Association* 233, no. 7 (2008).

10 Common Situations

Dealing with Emergencies and Crisis Situations

A client rushes into your pet hospital cradling Gus, her Labrador retriever beagle, in her arms. It seems that Gus was hit by a car—he slipped through the fence while the client was across the street visiting a neighbor. Gus's injuries are severe and his life is in danger. You try to take Gus from her but she is clutching him to her chest and has launched into an emotional monologue describing her reactions to the accident. "He's such a good dog . . . I can't imagine ever losing him," she says over and over again. You realize that if she doesn't let go of Gus, he will die. It's time for you to take control of the situation.

Assessment: What's Going on Here?

Emergencies and crisis situations create some of the most complex and difficult interactions you will see in your professional life. During crisis situations, people tend to drop to lower levels of functioning and have more trouble communicating in general. The skills they normally use to cope with difficult situations seemingly no longer work or are forgotten. Typical characteristics and emotions of a person in crisis include the following:

- **Feeling out of control, panicked, and confused.** This creates an intense amount of anxiety that can affect everything the person in crisis thinks or expresses.
- **Feeling that the grief and sadness will be too much to bear**.
- **Physical disturbances** (shortness of breath, rapid heartbeat, or impairment of balance and motor coordination).
- **Experiencing distortions in time** (either events seem to move very quickly or time feels frozen).

- **Tunnel vision** (inability to consider more than one solution to a problem).
- **Difficulty recalling or remembering information.**

Plan
Communication Protocol: What to Do, What to Say

STEP 1   Lay the Foundation

Your first goal in an emergency situation like this is to stabilize the client so she can deal with what is going on *now*. This requires doing a quick assessment of her needs and finding out which issues can be dealt with later. In crises, it is helpful for a veterinary team to split up so each person can accomplish his or her individual tasks (the doctor and veterinary technician can provide emergency medical care while the client care specialist talks to the client). Other things to consider:

- **Create structure for the client.** This helps stabilize and calm her down. For the example above, you might gently yet firmly take Gus from the client's arms or ask her to carry Gus into the treatment area. Then immediately guide her into an exam room. This helps the client focus better and removes the involvement of other clients in the waiting room (sometimes during a crisis, bystanders attempt to help and inadvertently make the situation worse). Use concise language when asking clients to follow you or go somewhere with you.
- **Structure your physical environment in a way that fosters effective communication.** Comfortable, mobile chairs and an area with water or coffee help clients with their most pressing physical needs. Offering a chair, a tissue, or simply inviting them to sit down and breathe with you can help clients focus better and feel less scared. If a client has small children, ask her if you can provide the children with toys, books, or activities to keep them occupied.

STEP 2   Conduct the Communication

- **Use a soft and reassuring tone of voice to support, reassure, and calm clients down.** Acknowledge clients' emotions (this will reassure them that you really get what they're going through). Tell them that everything possible is being done to help their pet.
- **Give clients permission to think, feel, and behave however they need to (within safe limits).** You can empower your clients by encouraging them to ask for what they need or to make requests that are important to them. Encourage clients to use the telephone to contact someone who may be able to come and help them.
- **Be very specific and direct with your updates or instructions to the client.** For example, "I'm going to go back to the treatment area to get an update for you. I'll be back in a few minutes." Or, "Please walk with me to the front desk for a minute so you can use the telephone." Clients in crisis respond best to clear, concise words.
- **Involve the whole veterinary team to assist clients in finding outside resources of support and referrals.** Do this once you have gotten past the initial crisis.
- **Keep in mind that clients may be in a state of shock.** Make them aware of this before they drive or perform any other task. Encourage them to contact a friend or family member for support.

STEP 3   Stay Connected through Follow-Up Care

- **Follow up with your client with a phone call or another appointment when the crisis is over.** For your staff, try to debrief when possible (or write a note to yourself to discuss it at the next staff meeting).

When the News Is Bad: A Four-Step Process for Delivering Bad News

Many crisis situations may require you to deliver bad news (such as an animal's death or terminal condition). Many veterinary professionals feel anxious about doing this because delivering bad news can be both stressful and difficult. However, using a standard communication protocol will help you say what you need to say in the kindest, most direct way possible. It is best to think of delivering bad news as a series of four steps:

1. Prepare yourself emotionally for clients' potential responses, keeping in mind that they may be in an emotional crisis (shock, sadness, crying, anger, denial).
2. Tell clients that there is bad news that will be difficult for them to hear.
3. Deliver the bad news as clearly and concisely as possible. For example, "I'm sorry to tell you that despite all of our best efforts to save Gus, he has died. We tried to revive him with CPR for ten minutes but his injuries were just too extensive."
4. Give clients permission to express themselves by normalizing their feelings and using appropriate self-disclosure. For example, "It's okay to cry [be angry, upset, shocked, etc.]. I would cry too if my dog had died."

After the initial response to the news, explain it in more detail and discuss all of the necessary information. If the pet has died, refer to the protocol described in Situation 10 of this book, "Dealing with Grieving Clients." If you've just given a difficult diagnosis such as cancer or another life-threatening condition, ask the client if he would like to discuss treatment options now, or if he needs some time before proceeding. If the medical situation requires that the client make an immediate decision, validate this difficulty. For example, "This must be so hard for you, and it's unfair that you have to make this decision so quickly. I'm sorry that you can't have more time."

ROLE-PLAY IDEAS

For hospital managers/client care specialists: Use the situation described above and practice reassuring and calming the client. Practice your tone of voice, paying close attention to the verbal communication skills you will need in this situation.

For veterinary technicians: Use this same situation and practice how you might provide periodic updates to the client. You can also practice delivering bad news using the protocol described here.

For veterinarians: Practice delivering bad news. Pay attention to your tone of voice, word choice, and demeanor. Practice making a referral.

Your Notes

Dealing with Financial Constraints

A client arrives at your hospital with her six-month-old Siberian husky puppy, Juno. She tells you that she adopted Juno right after a bad breakup with her boyfriend, and that Juno has always been there for her. You discover that Juno has a parvovirus infection and that the prognosis is fairly good, but only if you can pursue aggressive treatment right away. Treatment requires at least two to three days of hospitalization. You give the client a price estimate and she begins to cry, telling you that she can't possibly afford the treatment. She says that she's badly in debt and appeals to you to "help save her baby."

Assessment: What's Going on Here?

Discussing money and the cost of veterinary services presents a challenge to most veterinary teams. The issue of money is particularly difficult because it almost always involves high levels of emotion as well as life-and-death situations for the animal. *Financial issues are almost inevitably paired with the perception of care and compassion.* This is unfortunate because no one can put a price tag on compassion.

The difficult setup for veterinary professionals is that many people measure your level of compassion in a monetary way. In addition, many pet owners have unrealistic ideas and expectations about the cost of veterinary services. The average pet owner does not appreciate and understand all that is involved in quality veterinary care. In fact, some pet owners do not even know how much education, time, and training you have invested in becoming a veterinary professional.

Many pet owners think of veterinary care in the same financial terms as they do their own medical care—care that is usually covered by their insurance company. As a result, many people have little appreciation for the true costs of human medical services. For example, they might make a $10 to $20 copayment or pay 20 percent for a surgery that costs thousands of dollars (it's hard for clients to understand why a radiograph for their cat costs $50 to $100 when a radiograph of their own foot costs them only a $20 co-payment). Since insurance is still uncommon in veterinary medicine, pet owners pay the full price of services without really understanding what a great value it is. A similar procedure or surgery in veterinary medicine is usually a fraction of the cost it would be in human medicine.

Another factor is a simple lack of education or planning. Some people buy or adopt animals impulsively without thinking through all the financial consequences. Still others have little understanding about the medical needs of their animals and find themselves unprepared when problems arise.

The truth is that all veterinary professionals face financial situations that will frustrate them, challenge them, and tug at their heartstrings. You may end up euthanizing a pet you'd really prefer to treat, or watch a client leave your hospital upset and frustrated. The best way to help clients with financial limits is to communicate as openly, honestly, and compassionately as possible.

Plan
Communication Protocol: What to Say, What to Do

STEP 1   Lay the Foundation

- **Educate your clients.** Your most valuable tool in dealing with financial issues is client education. If you can find the extra fifteen minutes, you can often answer your client's money-based questions and explain the cost of her animal's care. When discussing money, it is important for you to expect that your client may have high emotions, and you should be adequately prepared to deal with them.
- **Determine ahead of time if money issues will be a personal hook for you.** For many veterinarians it is. If you know ahead of time how you might potentially react to these situations, you will be adequately prepared to deal with them when they arise. *The key is to uncouple your*

sense of compassion from your responsibility to your business and providing good medical care.

- **Don't undercharge.** You cannot possibly provide quality medical care if you are constantly undercharging for your services. Remind yourself that having a commitment to your business, employer, or your family's financial well-being does not mean that you do not love animals. You, and possibly your employer, will determine if and when there are special circumstances under which you might discount or provide complimentary veterinary services.

STEP 2   Conduct the Communication

- **Set limits ahead of time.** Make your payment policy clear at the very beginning of the appointment to avoid misunderstandings later on.
- **Validate and acknowledge your client's reaction to financial limitations.** Be aware that the client may be feeling scared, shocked, embarrassed, angry, or guilty about not being able to afford veterinary services. Whenever possible, say, "It must be frightening to realize how much effort it is going to take to treat Biscuit. I know that his illness is a real shock to you." Or, "I can see that you really want to help Kelsey, but you are surprised by the cost of this surgery. You obviously care for her very much and were not expecting this sudden expense."
- **Depersonalize your clients' comments if they get angry.** When clients vent their frustration, it is usually more about them than it is about you. Some clients can become desperate and may appeal to your sense of guilt by asking, "Don't you care about animals?" In these situations, it is helpful to make the client understand that your financial limitations do not reflect your level of compassion any more than they do for them. "I know how much you love Sunshine. I care about her too. However, just as your financial constraints do not reflect how much you love her, my commitment to her cannot be judged by my own financial limitations. I'd like to see if we can work together and find some options that will allow us both to help Sunshine the best way that we can, given both our financial needs."
- **Use self-disclosure to let clients know that you do understand and care.** "Finances are one of the toughest parts of my job. I do this work

because I love animals. I feel sad and frustrated when I can't help them for free."

- **Educate clients about your costs.** Demonstrate the procedures you performed. "It sounds like you have some concerns about your bill. We're dedicated to providing quality health care for Otter, and unfortunately that caliber of care quickly adds up. Would you like me to show you some of what we did and talk about the services that we provided for him today?"

- **Provide written information and estimates** for the medical procedures you perform and prepare the client for possible future expenses. Have clients sign the estimates in advance and provide a range for the potential costs involved with a particular medical procedure. Allow for a cushion when you give a price range but don't overestimate too much.

- **Explore other options.** Try to keep the client the responsible party when figuring out how to pay for an animal's treatment. Alternatives might include using "Care Credit" or some other company that can help clients with financial constraints, finding family or friends who will lend your client a credit card, getting an advance on a paycheck, or even borrowing the money from someone else (instead of from you!).

STEP 3 — Stay Connected Through Follow-Up Care

If the financial limitations were successfully resolved, schedule a call to the client as a way to check up afterward. This reminds clients of the good value they're receiving. Also, it is important to keep in mind that financial issues can be very emotional and stressful for the entire veterinary staff. You can address some of these issues by using creative alternatives such as these:

- **Donate a small percentage of profits to create a general client subsidy fund.** Some veterinary practices create special funds for unusual circumstances like animal abuse or emergencies. Employees can donate to these funds, and clients who might want to memorialize an animal in a special way can give a gift in its name. Clients like the idea of helping other animals and owners who are in financial need.

- **Promote pet health insurance.**

- **Be consistent, both personally and in your practice.** When you do reduce a fee or give away your services, be aware that there may be consequences. People talk. You might feel terrific after financially helping

Mrs. Brown save her little beagle, but you may have more problems that you expected when the women in Mrs. Brown's church group do not understand why you can't do the same for their pets.

- **Remember to believe in the value of your services.** You have worked very hard and put forth a substantial financial investment to obtain your degree and level of training. You provide a valuable service and deserve to be compensated for those services. Remembering this will help you to separate your sense of compassion from your financial responsibilities and help you to deal with emotional conversations involving money.

ROLE-PLAY IDEAS

For hospital managers/client care specialists: Role-play the situation above and practice communicating with clients in all the various ways clients might respond to money issues.

For veterinary technicians: Practice how you would educate a client about a pet's treatment and the costs involved.

For veterinarians: Practice this scenario using skills that will help you set limits, educate effectively, and be compassionate. Take notice of how you are feeling in these situations. Do you feel guilty, sad, or frustrated? This will help you recognize and work through your own personal hooks.

Your Notes

Dealing with Mistakes, Accidents, or Unexpected Outcomes

Your clients have chosen cremation for their dog, Comet, after he dies. They wish to have Comet individually cremated, with the remains (ashes) returned to them afterward. Since your clinic offers this service to clients, you agree to make the appropriate arrangements with the local pet cemetery/crematory.

After a week, you realize that Comet's cremated remains have not come back to your office. After speaking with the people at the crematory and checking back through your own records, you realize that you forgot to write down your clients' request for individual cremation. The pet crematory's policy is that, without written instructions designating a body for individual cremation, all bodies are taken care of by mass cremation, with the ashes scattered on the grounds of the pet cemetery. The sick feeling in your stomach tells you that this is what happened to Comet.

You're concerned about protecting yourself. What if your clients take their business to another clinic or, even worse, decide to sue you? That afternoon, the clients swing by unexpectedly to pick up Comet's cremated remains. You now have to explain to them what has happened.

Assessment: What's Going on Here?

Some people refuse to apologize, even when they know they are clearly wrong, because they don't want to feel like they're in a vulnerable position. For them being vulnerable usually feels like a loss of power or strength.

Some people blame others when mistakes are made. Blaming is a way to shirk responsibility. Psychologists say we blame others for things we've done because we are afraid of rejection, afraid that people will think less of us if they find out what we've done. Still others apologize and take responsibility for everything that goes wrong, even when they are clearly *not* responsible. None of these attitudes are effective ways to communicate or to rectify mistakes.

Being honest goes hand in hand with apologizing. In some cases, offering an apology also means taking responsibility and attempting to right a wrong. When you decide to be honest and to apologize to a client, it is an opportunity to use every communication technique described in this book. While apologizing and being honest are almost always the professional and right thing to do, it still takes tremendous courage for you to do so.

Plan
Communication Protocol: What to Say, What to Do

STEP 1   Lay the Foundation

- **Structure your environment** so you have a quiet, private, comfortable place to talk.

STEP 2   Conduct the Communication

- **Acknowledge your mistake** and deliver the news in a sensitive way (use the suggested strategies for delivering bad news in Situation 1).
- **Use active listening and paraphrasing** to understand your clients' responses and current requests.
- **Be immediate with your own feelings.** Self-disclose about your sadness and regret.
- **Finally, be as honest as possible.** Use the previous example: "When Comet died, I said I would be responsible for making the arrangements to have him cremated. After you left, I filled out the form for the crematory, but I neglected to note your wishes concerning individual cremation and the return of Comet's ashes. As a result, Comet was part of a mass cremation and I am unable to give you his individual cremated remains. I sincerely apologize. I am so sorry I made this mistake."

STEP 3   Stay Connected Through Follow-Up Care

Your honesty and willingness to apologize will pay off in cases where your clients forgive you and remain loyal to your practice. However, even if you encounter clients who refuse to forgive you and take their business elsewhere, it's important for you to acknowledge that there is personal success in simply doing the right thing, regardless of the outcome. Congratulations!

ROLE-PLAY IDEAS

For hospital managers/client care specialists: Role-play the situation above and practice apologizing. Pay close attention to your verbal and nonverbal skills. Also try a role-play where the client is surprised by an unexpected outcome.

For veterinary technicians: Practice apologizing to clients by using your communication skills. Do the same with unexpected outcomes.

For veterinarians: Practice apologizing to clients about a mistake or accident. Role-play a situation where the client is upset about an unexpected outcome (like an adverse reaction to a vaccination). Use the four-step plan for delivering bad news (presented in Situation 1).

Your Notes

Dealing with Angry Clients

A client calls about his dog, who recently had surgery. Suddenly he explodes with "I'm not going to pay a cent for this surgery! Wally is sicker now than when I first brought him in to see you. I wonder if any of you know what you're doing around here. You don't appear to give a damn about him at all!"

Assessment: What's Going on Here?

Anger is a normal, natural emotion that all people feel from time to time. What makes anger so difficult for most people to deal with is the negative energy behind it. If you work to understand why your client is angry, you have a much better chance at diffusing it. The key is to stay calm and try to keep the situation under control.

Remember that as a care provider, you are in a position of power because the pet owner needs or wants something from you (a healthier pet, reassurance, and understanding). If the client realizes that being angry or yelling at you will not help him to get what he wants, the anger will usually lessen.

Some common reasons why pet owners become angry are:

- **Finances:** an inability to pay or unrealistic expectations about the cost of veterinary services.
- **Treatment complications and unexpected problems.**
- **Dissatisfaction with services:** the perception that their animal has been mishandled or mistreated in some way.
- **Time conflicts:** unrealistic expectations about treatment times, being kept waiting.
- **Poor communication:** minor misunderstandings, unresolved conflicts.

- **Lack of information or preparation:** feeling inadequately prepared to deal with a pet's illness (physical appearance, financial issues, etc.).
- **Lack of continuity of care:** seeing a different veterinary professional during each visit, feeling "passed around."
- **Emotional responses to an animal's illness or death:** Use anger as a mask for other emotions they are feeling as a result of a pet's illness or death; anger is sometimes expressed because it is the easiest and least threatening emotion to access.
- **Masking other emotions with anger:** feeling helpless or powerless, fear, guilt, sadness, and grief.

There are, of course, times when another person's anger is abusive or completely inappropriate. In these situations, your job is to protect yourself and other members of the staff. Your responsibility as a care provider never extends to remaining in a place or near a person that is abusive or potentially dangerous. It is also important to develop and maintain good self-care skills when confronted with angry clients. Remember that you are not responsible for the way in which clients express their anger, and you can only do your best in responding to them with openness and sincerity. Being around angry people can be very draining. Remind yourself that there is more to your life than just work, and take the extra time to participate in activities and hobbies that you enjoy outside of work.

Plan
Communication Protocol: What to Say, What to Do

STEP 1   Lay the Foundation

- **Know your own response to anger.** Some people freeze up when confronted with intense anger, while others tend to strike back. Know your own "anger buttons" and be aware of how and when clients might push those buttons. Take a few deep breaths to calm your body and gain composure. While you are breathing, think about ways that you can *respond* to the anger rather than *react* to it.
- **Move your discussion to a private place.** Structure your environment so you can calmly speak face-to-face.

STEP 2 Conduct the Communication

- **Don't get defensive.** The majority of people who are angry just want to be heard and understood. A client's anger is usually more about his own frustrations or problems than it is about you. If you take it personally and lose your cool, you will only escalate the level of anger. Help the person regain control, and model this by staying in control yourself. Remember that, in any interaction, the more relaxed individual is also the more powerful.

- **Let your client vent.** Once a client has blown off steam, he can more easily discuss the issue rationally.

- **Validate your client's feelings and experiences as much as you honestly can.** Self-disclosure is often a good way to do this. For example, "I can see that you are very angry about Wally's progress. I can tell that you love him a lot and it must be so frustrating to see him feeling so poor. I am frustrated too and want to help him. Would you be willing to meet with me so we can discuss your concerns more thoroughly?"

- **Use open-ended questions to understand your client's needs, complaints, and concerns.** "I know Spicer is important to you. I want what is best for her too. What specifically is it that you need today?"

- **Communicate empathy and apologize if appropriate.** "I can see that you are very angry about the delay. We've had quite a busy day and I'm sorry that you had to wait. Can we talk for a few minutes about Snowball's surgery?"

- **Set limits regarding your client's behavior and the kind of communication you will not tolerate.** "I want to help you with Midas and want to hear your concerns, but I can't help you while you are yelling at me." Or, "I'd like to help but I won't if you continue to insult me."

- **Use gentle confrontation and paraphrasing to help your client explore deeper feelings beneath the anger.** This works best with clients you know quite well and with whom you have an established foundation of trust. "I understand you are very angry about Barney's death. I also get the sense that your feelings of sadness run very deep and are causing you great pain. It's sad to lose such a wonderful friend. Sometimes anger is a part of grief. I wonder if you're just plain angry about the fact that Barney died."

STEP 3   Stay Connected Through Follow-Up Care

- Schedule a call with angry clients you have successfully dealt with.
- **Sometimes, despite your best efforts, you cannot diffuse a client's anger by yourself (or at all).** If you're unable to calm the client, ask someone else on the staff to join you or refer the client to a colleague for assistance. If the client becomes abusive or completely inappropriate, calmly yet firmly ask him to leave.

ROLE-PLAY IDEAS

For hospital managers/client care specialists: Role-play a situation in which a client wants you to diagnose a pet's problem on the phone. Practice explaining why you can't do this while acknowledging the client's anger/frustration about having to bring the pet in (and pay an examination fee).

For veterinary technicians: Practice telling a client that you cannot make a diagnosis about a particular illness or issue. Acknowledge his or her anger about having to wait for the veterinarian to get solid answers. Practice responding to a verbal attack such as "If a veterinary technician can't diagnose an illness, what exactly are you here for?"

For veterinarians: Role-play a client who is angry that your particular treatment plan is not yet helping. Practice responding to a client who attacks your medical knowledge and competence.

Your Notes

_____

_____

_____

_____

_____

Dealing with Client Complaints

A client calls in and sounds upset and angry. Finally she says, "I'm very disappointed in the way Winston was treated at your hospital. When I brought him home, he had a foul odor and looked tired. He was upset for two whole days, and I had a difficult time coaxing him out from under the bed."

Assessment: What's Going on Here?

As with many other professionals who provide services to the public, there are times when you must deal with client complaints and demands. Even though your profession is about medicine, you are still in a business that requires customer satisfaction. In veterinary medicine, client complaints and demands can range from the predictable and expected to the outrageous and unreasonable. Many factors can determine how demanding or satisfied a given client will be. These include client personality, client expectations (realistic vs. unrealistic), the bond between the client and the animal, and the client's perceptions of veterinary care.

Complaints and demands are a regular part of your practice. The key is how you respond to these situations. Your most powerful tool is your ability to communicate well with your clients. If you can do this, you will save yourself lots of time and tons of frustration.

Plan
Communication Protocol: What to Say, What to Do

STEP 1   Lay the Foundation

- **Respect the clients' privacy.** Move the conversation to a private space where you and your client can sit down together comfortably.
- **Recognize that complaining or demanding clients may be highly bonded to their animals and feeling very anxious or worried about them.** Take time to determine the exact nature of your clients' needs, problems, complaints, or concerns.
- **Be proactive.** You can often prevent client complaints by providing good client education. For instance, you should always prepare clients for any potential complications, problems, appearances, or behaviors that might be of concern after a medical procedure or surgery. Using the scenario at the beginning of this situation, you might say, "When we bring Winston to you I want you to be aware that he will look differently than when you left him here yesterday. He has an incision on his belly that is about three inches long. We shaved the fur around this area and there is a bandage covering the incision. This area might be red and swollen for a day or two. He might also smell a bit funny from the anesthesia and have some spots on his fur. Also, he might not be his usual bouncy self for a few days. This is normal after a surgery and will give him time to rest and recuperate. I have written down some instructions for you on how to take care of him and what to look for if there are complications. If you think of any other concerns, please call us during our office hours and we'll be glad to help you."

STEP 2   Conduct the Communication

- **Use open-ended questions** to determine what is motivating the client to complain or to be demanding, like the following:
  1. "What is your biggest concern at this point?"
  2. "What could we have done differently?"
  3. "Can you tell me more about what you're thinking or feeling?"
  4. "How can I best support you through this?"
  5. "Where would you like to go from here?"

- **Acknowledge your clients' complaints** and invite them to discuss them with you further. Don't get defensive in response, but rather open the lines of communication by actively listening to what they have to say. You can then evaluate whether or not the complaint seems justified or unreasonable. "I hear that you are very concerned about Winston and want him to have the very best care possible. Let's go over your concerns one by one and see if we can clear up any doubts that you may have regarding the care he received."
- **If the complaint seems justified, you may want to apologize** and adjust your care to fit the client's needs. Letting your client know your view as to the cause of the misunderstanding may also be useful. "I'm sorry you had to wait an hour past your scheduled appointment today. We had an emergency this morning that needed our immediate attention in order to save the animal's life. We appreciate your patience. And in the future we will notify you of changes in our appointment schedules. As for today, would you like me to examine Buddy now or would you like to reschedule?"
- **If the complaint seems unreasonable, acknowledge the client's feelings** while setting limits and providing client education. "I can see that you had hoped to be seen immediately today and that you are concerned about Casey. Unfortunately, we can't always respond to a walk-in appointment right away. Since Casey's condition isn't critical, I need to see the four other clients who had scheduled appointments first. Either I can see you and Casey as soon as I'm finished with them or you can make an appointment with the receptionist for another time."

Overly demanding clients may have unrealistic expectations. Ask questions that will help you to determine how realistic their expectations are, such as "What are your expectations of me and of our staff?" or "What is your goal in coming here today?" Or you might say, "I can see that you had different ideas about how your appointment with Misty would go today. Let me share with you how our hospital works and answer any questions that you might have to see if we can meet your needs."

- **Always acknowledge the bond between the animal and owner.** Ask your client to work with you to address the complaint. "I know that you are unhappy at this point and I'm not sure if we're getting anywhere. It's so obvious to me that Winston is very important to you and it's important to me that you and Winston receive quality care. Can you help me figure out what we could do together to resolve our differences and continue to help Winston?" Pet owners can feel scared and powerless when their animals become sick, especially when they don't have the power to make their loved ones feel better. Therefore, they look to you to help them. In order to allow you to help their pet, they must withdraw their own control and place their trust in you. This can make owners feel very vulnerable. A person attempting to cope with feelings of fear and helplessness can become very demanding or critical.

How to Handle Unreasonable Client Expectations and Set Boundaries

- Acknowledge your client's need or request and clearly establish your limits. "I understand it's difficult to ask for time away from your job; however, I don't make appointments during the evening hours."
- Use self-disclosure to solidify or to justify (if you feel you need to) your limits. "As I said, I don't make evening appointments. I have a spouse and two young children who are my priorities after work."
- Say no to the request you cannot grant, but offer a compromise. "I can't see you at seven o'clock at night, but you can drop Pepper off before eight a.m. and pick him up at five p.m. We'll treat him and care for him while you're at work."
- If the client persists, use immediacy or gentle confrontation to repeat your "no" answer and maintain your boundaries. "You and Pepper are important to me, and I respect the fact that you need to make arrangements to have Pepper treated at a time when it won't interfere with your job. However, I'm beginning to feel frustrated with your unwillingness to understand and accommodate my schedule."
- Provide your client with written materials stating your clinic's policies regarding treatment schedules, appointment hours, after-hours emergency fees, and so on.

Sometimes complaining about your services or demanding special treatment is a way for clients to test you (get your attention, regain some control). They might deduce that, if you are able to handle their complaints and meet every demand they throw at you, you are probably also capable of successfully treating their companion animal. Most clients don't consciously decide to behave this way. Rather, their complaints and demands are unconscious reactions to their feelings of anxiety. While it's true that most clients cannot accurately assess your medical skills, they can certainly assess your communication skills. Thus, you can mitigate a lot of complaints and demands by simply acknowledging your clients' feelings and gently reassuring them that you care.

STEP 3   Stay Connected Through Follow-Up Care

- **Schedule a call for the clients** and check on the status of their complaint. Answer any questions and invite them to call back if they want.
- **Work together.** You and your coworkers must be a team when it comes to working with overly demanding clients. It's important to ensure that you are all communicating the same message. Be careful to set limits up front and don't let clients split your staff. For example, if one member of your staff gets intimidated and bends the rules to accommodate a demanding client, it will be difficult for someone else to set limits later on and enforce clinic policies. Remember to work together to try to meet your clients' needs while also supporting one another. Staff meetings are excellent times to deal with these issues.

ROLE-PLAY IDEAS

For hospital managers/client care specialists: Think about some of the most demanding clients at your hospital. Use a role-play to act out how you would deal with them. Focus on client education and use open-ended questions to guide you.

For veterinary technicians: Practice doing a follow-up appointment or a bandage change following a procedure or surgery. Have the client complain about a whole host of things. Practice responding and educating the client about his or her complaints without getting defensive.

For veterinarians: Role-play a situation in which the client expects to hear from you on an unreasonable time schedule. Try setting limits and describing your point of view. Educate the client and practice talking about differing expectations.

Your Notes

Dealing with Anxious Clients

You try to take a cat to the back for a normal procedure but the pet's owner protests, "Why can't I go into the back treatment room with you and hold Dugan while you take care of him? I don't want to leave him right now. He gets very scared when I'm not with him."

Assessment: What's Going on Here?

Clients may be anxious and even suspicious of your motives for a variety of reasons. For instance, their hesitancy may be based on a previous negative experience or simply be the result of a collection of life experiences. When it comes to the health and well-being of a beloved companion animal, though, anxiety may become exaggerated, especially about medical or surgical procedures that nonmedical people don't understand.

When pet owners entrust you with the care and well-being of their animals, they often perceive themselves to be powerless. This feeling of helplessness, paired with a lack of control over their pet's situation, can create anxiety or fear that results in distrust.

Plan
Communication Protocol: What to Say, What to Do

STEP 1 Lay the Foundation

The most effective way to deal with anxious clients is to establish trust and rapport early. Trust is confidence or a belief in someone's goodness and integrity. Rapport is a harmonious and useful relationship or communication. Trust and rapport are the cornerstones of effective communication.

STEP 2 Conduct the Communication

- **Self-disclose with casual conversation** to find common ground. Some people are intimidated by professionals, especially doctors, and seeing you as an ordinary human being with the same interests and concerns as they have will help them relax.
- **Normalize your clients' concerns or uneasiness.** "When I take my children to the pediatrician, I have a hard time leaving them alone. It's so hard when you're worried about someone you love."
- **Touch and talk to your clients' animals.** The quickest way to your clients' collective heart is to demonstrate that you have a sincere liking for and interest in their pets.
- **Use immediacy if the client appears unusually anxious.** "I realize that we've just met and that you don't know me very well. I also realize that you are uncomfortable leaving Klondike here and seem very concerned about the care he'll receive. Can you help me understand why you feel that way? Has something happened that I should be aware of?"
- **Communicate warmth and sincerity with your words and nonverbal behavior.** Be open and approachable and use active listening, paraphrasing, direct eye contact, and open body posture. Always handle your clients' animals gently and their feelings compassionately.
- **Maintain your clients' confidentiality.** Unless you have permission to discuss a case, anything of a personal nature that your client confides in you must be kept between the two of you.
- **Perform procedures in the exam room in the client's presence whenever possible.**

STEP 3 Stay Connected Through Follow-Up Care

- **Be patient.** Trust and rapport usually develop naturally over time, but they can be enhanced with some simple techniques. In building trust and rapport, patience is important. Some clients will automatically distrust you without any legitimate or rational reason. Try not to get defensive or to take it personally. Their lack of trust probably has little to do with you and more to do with their own experiences with the veterinary medical community in general. Some people who have had negative experiences with professionals in human medicine will transfer feelings to you.

- **Show interest in your clients' personal lives.** "The last time you were here with Scooter, you were adding a new addition to your house. How is that going?"
- **Compliment clients on how they care for their companion animals.** "Scotty has lost weight since the last time I've seen him! I remember that we talked about his diet and the trouble with feeding him table scraps. You told me how hard it was for you to say no when he begged, but you've done an excellent job at following through with the recommendations. That's great."
- **Encourage clients to ask questions.** Many people are naturally apprehensive about medical procedures of which they have little knowledge. It is important for you to take the initiative here because many people will not tell you when they don't understand the meaning of complex medical information. Clients may even nod their head and appear to understand because they don't want to look foolish or ignorant in front of you.

ROLE-PLAY IDEAS

For hospital managers/client care specialists: Role-play a situation using some of your most anxious clients as a blueprint. Practice reassuring the client and addressing the client's fears.

For veterinary technicians: Practice dealing with a client who tends to be reassured by the doctor only. Use your verbal and nonverbal skills to convey a sense of trust and deal with the client's anxiety.

For veterinarians: Role-play a client who demands to follow you to the back treatment area to watch you and your staff treating his or her pet. Discuss times when you might allow this request and other times when it would be inappropriate.

Your Notes

Dealing with Indecisive Clients

A client sits across from you in the exam room, going back and forth about the next step. She says, "I just don't know if I should go ahead with Max's surgery. I know that it's risky to do it, but I also know that it is Max's only real chance. I don't think I'm ready to let him go yet without trying something, but I'm just so confused. I simply can't make a decision. What would you do if Max were your dog?"

Assessment: What's Going on Here?

Pet owners often face difficult decisions. Clients who care deeply for their animals often struggle with decisions about procedures like surgery, amputation, chemotherapy, and euthanasia. Since companion animals are almost completely dependent upon their owners for their care and well-being, many owners feel that they have made unspoken contracts with their animals to love and take care of them. This sense of responsibility can create great emotional distress for owners when they believe that their animals are trusting them with their lives and well-being.

Plan

Communication Protocol: What to Say, What to Do

STEP 1 Lay the Foundation

- **With indecisive clients, the single most important thing to discuss is the issue of quality of life for the animal.** This will give you and the client a common reference point and a way of structuring your interaction. Different clients have different standards for quality of life and may define it in unique ways, according to the individual personality of the owner and the animal. Your job is to help clients identify what quality of life means for their animals and to communicate that you understand this. This might mean accepting a definition for quality of life that is somewhat different from your own.

- **Structure the environment and remove time barriers.** If there is no medical reason to require an immediate decision, structure the environment (give your client access to a private room and a telephone so she can consult with friends or family members) and remove time barriers so she can take several hours or even days to make the decision. "It seems like you're not 100 percent sure about your decision. Since there is no medical reason to rush, would you like to take Max home and give yourself some more time to prepare?"

STEP 2   Conduct the Communication

Indecisiveness usually stems from anxiety and a need to make the "right" decision. During decision making, then, your goal is to help clients realize that there may not be a right decision, only a decision that is right for them. The other part of your job is to lower your clients' anxiety about the decision-making process, normalizing their feelings within the context of their love for their animal. For example, "I can see how difficult this decision is for you. You want to give Max every chance possible, yet there are no guarantees. The fact is that what I might do for Max if he were my dog and what you might choose to do could be very different. There really is no right or wrong answer here. The most important thing for you to know is that whichever decision you make, I'll support you all the way."

- **Normalize your client's feelings and self-disclose, if appropriate.** "I know how much Max means to you and I can tell what a difficult decision this is for you. I would be struggling as much as you are if I were in your shoes."
- **Acknowledge your client's unique relationship with her companion animal.** "You and Max have a very special relationship and you are the expert on what is best for him. I can give you my medical opinion, but the fact is, I don't know him and understand him the way that you do."
- **Give your client permission to feel anxious and reframe it as a positive trait.** "Given how much you love Max, I'd be worried about you if

you weren't struggling with this decision. The fact that you are having trouble making a decision about his surgery is a sign of how much you truly care about him and want what is best."

- **Once a decision has been made, paraphrase your client's words and feelings to ensure you are both committed to the same course of action.** "It sounds like you want to proceed with Max's surgery. I understand that you feel anxious about it, and I also hear that you feel you would not forgive yourself if you did not give Max this chance. Am I hearing you correctly?"

STEP 3   Stay Connected Through Follow-Up Care

Whenever possible, check in with clients later on. Paraphrase their feelings and concerns. If they are still unable to make a decision, some other helpful decision-making techniques are these:

- **Ask if clients need more medical information.** "Would it be helpful if we reviewed the surgery once again and discussed the potential side effects?"
- **Help clients look at future consequences and potential circumstances.** "When you look back on this six months from now, what will be most important about what you did or did not do? Which decisions will be the easiest for you to live with? I believe it's part of my job to help you make decisions now that will minimize your regrets later on."
- **Encourage clients to talk with their animals.** Many owners have very special relationships with their pets. When tough decisions need to be made, you can encourage your clients to enlist their pet's help with decisions. "You and Max have always been able to communicate with each other. That is still the case now. Spend some time with Max, talk to him, and maybe he will be able to tell you what he wants. Because of how strongly connected the two of you are, I believe that you will come to the answer that is right for you together."
- **Be open to discussing euthanasia as an option if the medical status of the animal warrants it.** Be aware that clients might not want to pursue treatment but may be hesitant to tell you, because they don't want to look like a bad or uncaring person. "We know that Max's cancer is quite advanced. We've discussed options for treatment, but I want you to know that euthanasia is also an option. Doing every possible

treatment for Max is not necessarily proof of how much you love him. Looking at his quality of life is also a sign of your love, and I want you to know that I will also support you with this decision if it's the one you come to."

ROLE-PLAY IDEAS

For hospital managers/client care specialists: Practice a role-play of a client who frequently changes his or her mind about a medical procedure. Focus on making the client aware of this and help the client to make a definite decision.

For veterinary technicians: Act out a situation in which an indecisive client keeps asking you questions that really need to be answered by the doctor. Practice communicating your limits while still supporting them.

For veterinarians: Role-play the scenario at the beginning of this situation. Help the client move through a decision-making process while offering support and understanding.

Your Notes

_____

_____

_____

_____

_____

_____

_____

_____

Dealing with Children

A little boy looks up at you and explains, "My mama says you're going to do an operation on Fred's stomach. Why are you doing that? What's going to happen to him? I'm scared and just want him to go home with us!"

Assessment: What's Going on Here?

Children can be challenging clients. There's no doubt that explaining medical issues to a child (especially euthanasia) can be tricky, depending upon the child's age. However, children can also be refreshing clients and ones you look forward to dealing with. In some ways, children are easier to deal with than adults because they don't usually have the same preconceived notions, biases, or cynicism that adults have.

Pets are important to children. They serve many roles and provide stable emotional support even when the child is in trouble or being punished. Pets can act as siblings, playmates, protectors, and even surrogate parents. The bonds that children form with pets are profound and should not be underestimated.

Plan
Communication Protocol: What to Say, What to Do

STEP 1 Lay the Foundation

It is important to remember that children often require different explanations regarding medical issues. A child's level of maturity and developmental age determine how complex you should be in your conversations.

- **Don't use euphemisms.** Children are very concrete thinkers (especially ages ten and under). They do not think abstractly and they tend to interpret what is said in very literal ways. For this reason, it is never a good idea to use euphemisms such as "The pet was put to sleep" when talking to a child. Instead, the goal should be to talk with the child openly and honestly using words and language that the child can understand.
- **Answer questions.** Children may have many questions for you and the entire veterinary team. Additionally, parents often look to you to set an example on what's best to say to the child.
- **Be aware of "magical thinking."** Young children often mistakenly believe that they are somehow responsible for the pet's well-being and that their thoughts and actions have the power to affect the pet's health. Make parents aware of this and encourage them to talk openly with their children.
- **Be honest.** Little white lies and euphemisms only frighten and confuse children (especially young children). Also encourage parents to be honest with their children about a pet's health and don't collude in lying to a child. Encourage parents to involve children as much as possible in decisions surrounding the pet's treatments, illnesses, and even death.

STEP 2   Conduct the Communication

Because euthanasia is the most difficult thing you will have to discuss with children, this step focuses on that. The death of a family pet is often a child's first experience with death and loss. It is an important time for parents and other adults to support children and teach them how to express grief in emotionally healthy ways, free of shame or embarrassment. Veterinarians can serve as a valuable resource for children during these times. Here are a few guidelines to follow:

- **Be as truthful as possible.** It's tempting to try to protect children from any kind of emotional pain. Yet attempting to soften the blow by telling children that a pet "ran away" or "went to live with someone else" only creates a different kind of pain. Losing a pet under any circumstances will cause children to grieve. Believing that a family pet ran away may make the grief worse by adding feelings of worry and abandonment.

- **Encourage children to view a pet's body and to say good-bye.** If a pet dies suddenly, it can be beneficial for children to see the pet's body and be able to say good-bye in whatever way they are comfortable with. This may include touching the pet, holding and hugging the pet, and even spending time alone with the pet's body. Depending on where the pet's death occurs, you or someone on your staff can clean the pet's fur of any blood, remove any medical equipment or supplies (catheters, tape, and so on), and position the body so it is soothing to see, perhaps curled into a pet bed or nestled into a container that has been lined with a soft blanket. Research, along with clinical experience, shows that it is beneficial for children to say a personal good-bye to a loved one who has died.

- **Involve children in the euthanasia process.** The key to a comforting good-bye process for children is *how well they are prepared to face their pet's death.* Encourage your clients to let their children talk to you and ask questions before a pet is euthanized. Children benefit from being well informed about the procedures they might witness. Children who are well prepared can usually handle the intense emotions that are part of euthanasia.

- **Allow children to make their own choices.** Whenever possible, children should be allowed to make their own choices about how much they wish to be involved in the process of saying good-bye to a pet. Older children may choose to be with a pet when the euthanasia is performed, while younger children may choose to say good-bye while their pet is still alive. Other children may choose to view a pet's body only after death has occurred, reassuring themselves that their beloved pet has really died. Very young children don't really understand death and have short attention spans. If a young child wants to be included in a euthanasia, it's a good idea for the parent to ask a friend to come along and take care of the child. This allows parents and older children uninterrupted time to say their own good-byes.

- **Allow time for grief.** Since children have shorter attention spans than adults and express their grief differently, be aware that they may grieve the loss in short bursts. Children are unable to sustain intense, grieving emotions for long periods of time. Therefore, it is normal for children to go from crying and being very upset one minute to wanting to go and play the next. This is not a sign of indifference or poor coping; it is simply the way in which children need to work through their grief.

STEP 3 Stay Connected Through Follow-up Care

- **Ask how the children are doing when you follow up with the parents.** This will impress parents and create an even deeper bond between you. Parents are reassured when they know that their children's well-being is important to you. This can create very loyal clients.

- **Determine whether children are unsupported in any of these areas.** If so, referrals to human service professionals are appropriate. Human service professionals might be teachers, school counselors, social workers, family therapists, members of the clergy, and counselors or support group facilitators who specialize in pet loss. It is wise to talk to human service professionals before referrals are made. Even though human service professionals may be highly qualified and skilled at what they do, they may not be trained to deal with grief or issues of pet loss.

- **Discuss the option.** It may be tempting for parents to try to cheer up grieving children by immediately adopting a new pet. Sometimes this works, and it is often at the children's own request. However, while some people are able to bond with a new pet and grieve for the one who died at the same time, there's no right time to adopt a new pet. Remind parents about how each family member is different. It's disturbing to children when the parent implies that a family member who dies is easily replaceable.

While adopting a new pet may help the whole family feel better, grieving together can also bring them closer together. Then, when everyone feels ready, a new pet can join the family and find his or her own joyful place in the home.

ROLE-PLAY IDEAS

For hospital managers/client care specialists: Have a staff member pretend to be a child who asks difficult and very direct questions about a pet's illness or death. Role-play situations in which you must talk to the parents as well.

For veterinary technicians: Practice talking to the child about medical issues and questions. Try out different language for different developmental ages.

For veterinarians: Role-play a situation where you must talk with the parent and the child about their pet's death or euthanasia. Have a staff member play a young child who asks very difficult questions and is difficult to talk with because he or she is very upset.

Your Notes

Dealing with Euthanasia Appointments

Casey Watson is a twelve-year-old golden retriever who has been diagnosed with lymphoma. Up to now chemotherapy has been effective, but now the cancer is back and more aggressive than ever. Casey's quality of life has deteriorated in the past few days and he is now refusing to eat or drink. The Watson family is coming in to euthanize Casey as your next appointment. The family consists of mother, father, ten-year-old son, and six-year-old daughter.

Assessment: What's Going on Here?

When clients have decided that euthanasia is the most loving and humane choice, it's important to remind them that they still have some control over when, where, and how the pet will die. It may feel strange or even morbid to "plan" a pet's death. However, remind your clients that the pet is going to die at some point—it is inevitable. The one last gift that clients can give a beloved friend is a peaceful, loving, painless death.

Plan
Communication Protocol: What to Say, What to Do

STEP 1 Lay the Foundation

- **Talk clients through the procedure,** educating them about what to expect and what drugs you will use. Be very specific and answer any questions they may have.

Encourage clients to stay with their pet during the euthanasia. Some clients will want to leave before the euthanasia; many want to stay but might be afraid that they will get emotional in front of you.

- **Work through the following euthanasia checklist** of questions with your clients:
  1. **When and where will it take place?** Do you want the procedure to be at home or do you feel comfortable going to the pet hospital? Where in the pet hospital can we go? Outside?
  2. **How will you take care of your pet's body?** Typical body care options include cremation (communal or private, burial in a pet cemetery or at home). Find out the details of each of these options beforehand so you can be prepared and select the option that is the most affordable and appropriate for you. Keep in mind that if you euthanize at a pet hospital and decide to bury your pet at home, you will need some way to carry the body home afterward.
  3. **Consider how you will want to say good-bye** to your companion. Who should be involved? Find out if special requests can be accommodated. In most situations they can be, but they may need to be prepared ahead of time. For example, some people like to recite special words, read poetry, play music, or say a prayer. This is your one and only chance to say good-bye. When you look back on this a year from now, what will be important for you to have done? Do you need to say something or do anything special before your pet's death?
  4. **Consider taking a memento of your pet.** A clay impression of a pet's paw makes a treasured memento. You might also consider taking a clipping of your pet's fur or a collar, tag, or other special objects. There are companies that sell products for pet mementos. These companies can be found in the "Resources" section of this book.
  5. **How will you take care of yourself** in the hours immediately following the euthanasia? Will it be safe for you to drive home (especially if you are alone)? You might consider taking the day off from work and being with friends and family who can support you after such an emotional experience.
- **Reassure clients** that it's normal to experience grief and that tears are completely acceptable.

STEP 2 Conduct the Communication

- **Let the client cry and hold the pet after the pet has been euthanized.** Though it is uncomfortable, silence is often the most appropriate thing.
- **When you do speak, make sure to continue acknowledging and normalizing the client's grief.**
- **Offer the client some privacy** with the pet for a specific time window. For example, "I'm going to step out and let you have a private moment. I will be back in about five minutes to check on you. If you want more time, please just let me know."

STEP 3 Stay Connected Through Follow-Up Care

- **Send a condolence card.** Give everyone on staff an opportunity to sign it (it should be sent within one week after the animal's death).
- **Update the client's records.**
- **Schedule a callback if you feel the need.** It may also be appropriate to provide outside grief resources and support to your client after the euthanasia (such as a pet loss support group, talking to a pet loss counselor, or visiting a particular website). By educating clients about grief, they will feel more comfortable in seeking out the support that is most helpful to them. You can also create some basic grief materials that describe the normal process of grief and help clients understand what is happening to them. Much of the information is included in Situation 10.

The most important thing to remember about euthanasia is that while you have been through many of these procedures before, it is often the very first time for the client. Remember the little details that communicate your sensitivity and concern.

ROLE-PLAY IDEAS

For hospital managers/client care specialists: Act out an entire euthanasia appointment from start to finish. Pay close attention to how you behave with the client and what you say.

For veterinary technicians: Role-play the entire euthanasia process and practice describing the procedure to a client. Be aware of both your verbal and nonverbal skills.

For veterinarians: Act out an entire euthanasia from start to finish, showing the rest of the staff what you say and what you do during this time. Many staff members are not in the exam room with clients when their animals are being euthanized. Educate your staff about your preferences and how you approach euthanasia.

Your Notes

_____

_____

_____

_____

_____

_____

_____

_____

_____

_____

_____

_____

_____

Dealing with Grieving Clients

After you diagnose your client's cat, she starts crying. She can't form her thoughts yet says, "I'm so sorry I'm crying. I shouldn't be this upset, and I'm embarrassed."

Assessment: What's Going on Here?

Crying is one of the classic nonverbal signs of grief. People cry when they are grieving because it is a natural reaction to emotional pain. Crying is an effective way to release emotion and an essential part of the grieving process. Still, like the client above, many people feel embarrassed or ashamed of their emotional outbursts.

Plan
Communication Protocol: What to Say, What to Do

STEP 1 Lay the Foundation

- **Don't worry if you get a little emotional too.** One of the biggest obstacles to connecting with grieving clients is probably your own fear that you will cry, too. It's not uncommon for veterinary professionals to abruptly end conversations with clients because they are afraid that they themselves will "lose control" in a professional situation.
- **Ensure that your clients have privacy**, along with tissues and a comfortable place to sit. This will give them permission to express their grief without fear of judgment or embarrassment.

STEP 2   Conduct the Communication

People generally feel better after crying and expressing grief. Grief counselors find that widows who had friends who encouraged them to cry were healthier than widows who experienced less encouragement from others to cry and to discuss their feelings of grief. It follows, then, that the best way to connect with your grieving clients is to encourage them to "get it out." Allow them to sob, wail, sniffle, and talk. If clients exhibit extreme displays of emotion, like panic attacks or sobbing, help them work through their waves of emotion.

Never leave the room because you *assume* your clients want to be alone. The act of leaving the room may signal your own embarrassment or disapproval of their grief. All forms of grieving (with the exception of responses that may be physically harmful to the client or to someone else) are healthy and acceptable forms of communication. Your job as a skilled communicator is to become comfortable with grief.

- **Acknowledge your client's grief.** "I can see how sad you are about Freddie's diagnosis."
- **Normalize your client's tears.** "I would expect you to cry in a situation like this."
- **Give permission to cry.** Offer your client a tissue and a place to sit down. "Take your time and let it out. I'm right here for you."
- **Touch the client if it seems appropriate.** Touch the client on places of the body that are neutral (such as the back of the shoulder, a light touch on the arm, or a quick hug if you know the client very well).
- **Self-disclose by crying yourself if you're moved to do so.** Crying demonstrates compassion and shows empathy for pets and their owners. "It's okay to cry. I cried when my dog died last year. It's perfectly normal to experience these emotions, and your tears show how much you loved your companion." If you cry easily you might say, "I often cry during times like this. I can still do my job, though, and be here for you." If you cry easily, you might also try switching your focus from what you are feeling to what you are thinking. In studies where researchers have asked people what they are crying about, people usually stop crying in order to think of an answer.

STEP 3 Stay Connected Through Follow-Up Care

- **Schedule a follow-up call** for the client to check in and see how she is doing. Make a referral for grief support if you feel it is appropriate.
- **Remember that your emotional responses to loss are normal,** too. Most clients feel comforted by their veterinarian's tears, but whether you cry or not, you may find it helpful to express your feelings or to take a few minutes for yourself to grieve in your own way. You will know you are dealing with patient death successfully when, instead of hardening yourself to the emotional ramifications of death, you allow yourself to actually feel the emotions that accompany loss and find ways to grieve.
- **Follow up and debrief** your staff about patient death (staff meetings can be a good time to do this). Allowing time for people to express their grief about a special patient in a supportive environment is essential to preventing compassion fatigue and burnout.

ROLE-PLAY IDEAS

For hospital managers/client care specialists: Practice by role-playing with a client who is unable to stop crying and feeling embarrassed by it. Pay close attention to what you say and what you communicate nonverbally.

For veterinary technicians: Practice by role-playing with a client who is crying and apologizing because of it. Practice using your nonverbal and verbal skills to offer support and normalize the client's feelings.

For veterinarians: Practice by role-playing with a client who is experiencing overwhelming grief. Use your nonverbal and verbal skills to respond to this client and practice making a grief referral afterward.

Your Notes

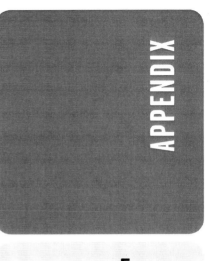

APPENDIX

Forms

Three-Step Emotional Support Protocol Planning Form

STEP 1   Lay the Foundation

- Prepare the physical environment.
- Stock client education/support supplies.
- Assign team member roles and responsibilities.

STEP 2   Conduct the Communication

- Establish trust and rapport.
- Use a variety of appropriate verbal and nonverbal clinical communication skills.
- Provide clients with educational/support products and information to take home.

STEP 3   Stay Connected Through Follow-Up Care

- Schedule a follow-up appointment or telephone call.
- Send a written communication (condolence card, thank-you note, etc.).
- Debrief case with staff members involved; role-play and review case at weekly staff meeting to improve everyone's communication knowledge and skills.

Sample Three-Step Emotional Support Protocol Planning Form

For Delivering Bad News

Before Your Case Begins

STEP 1 Lay the Foundation

- Prepare the physical environment.
  1. Prepare a private space with comfortable seating, tissues, information, etc.
  2. Assign roles and duties to staff members.
  3. Prepare yourself to deal with any response (shock, disbelief, anger, guilt, hysteria).
  4. Prepare clients.
     - Address them by name.
     - Prepare them for what is to come.
     - Predict how they may feel or respond: "Mrs. Brown, I have some bad news that may be upsetting for you to hear."
     - Stock client education/support supplies.
     - Assign team member roles and responsibilities.

During the Interaction

STEP 2 Conduct the Communication

- Establish trust and rapport.
  1. Give basic facts, telling clients of the death, illness, or injury up front. "We tried everything we knew how to do, but Max died during surgery. I want you to know he was anesthetized and felt no pain. We were all with him when he died."
  2. Be prepared to absorb the client's emotional response without becoming defensive, guilty, hurried, overly responsive, or offering intellectual explanations.

3. "I can imagine how hard this is."
4. "I know this is all overwhelming right now."
5. "We are really broken up about this, too."
6. "Would you like to spend some time with Max's body?"
- Use a variety of appropriate verbal and nonverbal clinical communication skills.
   1. Offer to provide more details now or at a later time.
   2. Help clients mobilize their personal support system by suggesting that they call a sympathetic friend or family member.
- Provide clients with educational/support products and information to take home.
   ° Offer to make a ClayPaws® print of Max's paw as a memorial to take with them.

After Your Client Leaves the Clinic

STEP 3 Stay Connected Through Follow-Up Care

- Schedule a follow-up appointment or telephone call.
   ° Call the next day to check on your client's well-being and to provide more information if requested.
- Send a written communication (condolence card, thank-you note, etc.).
   ° Send a condolence card and supportive information.
- Debrief case with staff members involved; role-play and review case at weekly staff meeting to improve everyone's communication knowledge and skills.

Role-Play Feedback Form

Name: _____ Date: _____

Role-play situation:

_____

_____

_____

_____

_____

Things that went well in the role-play:
(*to be filled out by colleagues observing the role-play*)

_____

_____

_____

_____

Ideas for improvement:
(*to be filled out by colleagues observing the role-play*)

_____

_____

_____

_____

Thank you for being willing to participate in this role-play. Your effort has helped all of us to learn! Great work!

Signed,

_____

Resources

Books for Professionals

Cornell, K., J. Brandt, and K. Bonvicini. "Effective Communication in Veterinary Practice." *Veterinary Clinics of North America: Small Animal Practice* vol. 37, no. 1 (January 2007).

Kurtz, S., J. Silverman, and J. Draper. *Teaching and Learning Communication Skills in Medicine*. Abingdon, Oxon, UK: Radcliffe Medical Press Ltd., 1998.

Lagoni, L. *The Practical Guide to Client Grief: Support Techniques for 15 Common Situations*. Lakewood, CO: AAHA Press, 1997.

Lagoni, L., C. Butler, and S. Hetts. *The Human-Animal Bond and Grief*. Philadelphia, PA: Saunders Company, 1994 (out of print).

Silverman, J., S. Kurtz, and J. Draper. *Skills for Communicating with Patients*. Abingdon, Oxon, UK: Radcliffe Medical Press Ltd., 1998.

Tannen, D. *Talking from 9 to 5: Women and Men at Work*. New York: Avon Books, 1994.

Client Information Products

World by the Tail, Inc.
"Caring for people who care for pets."
www.veterinarywisdom.com; info@wbtt.com
Offers products and services to foster veterinary-family communication and emotional support. Creators and distributors of ClayPaws®, the original paw print kit™, Veterinary Wisdom® products, and the Veterinary Wisdom® Resource Center.

Communication Skills Training

Argus Institute, Colorado State University, James L. Voss Veterinary Teaching Hospital
www.argusinstitute.colostate.edu; argus@colostate.edu
Offers bond-centered curriculum, clinical service for grief support, pet hospice program, and FRANK: Veterinarian-Client Communication Initiative (workshops and training with CE credits available).

Dana Durrance, MA

Veterinary Grief Specialist and Consultant

dldurrance@msn.com

Offers consulting and instruction services on various communication issues found in veterinary medicine. Speaking engagements, in-house training, and online consultation services.

Institute for Healthcare Communication, Inc.

info@healthcarecomm.org

A nationally accredited, not-for-profit organization that trains physicians and, in recent years, veterinarians throughout North America in effective communication skills. The veterinary communication training initiative is funded by a grant from Bayer Animal Health.

Professional Organizations

American Association for Human-Animal Bond Veterinarians (AAH-ABV)

http://aah-abv.org/net/home

Provides education, research, and support to enhance veterinarians' ability to create positive and ethical relationships among people, animals, and their environments.

Association for Veterinary Family Practice (AVFP)

www.avfp.org

Offers online and on-site (UC-Davis) coursework in the emerging specialty of veterinary family practice. Topics include pets in families and society and the clinical skills needed to care for both patients and clients.

Delta Society

"The human-animal health connection."

www.deltasociety.org

Improves human health through service and therapy animals.

International Conference on Communication in Veterinary Medicine (ICCVM)

www.iccvm.com; iccvm@bayleygroup.com

Promotes the development of veterinary communication research and education.

International Society for Anthrozoology (ISAZ)

www.isaz.net

Promotes the scientific and scholarly study of human-animal interactions. Also publishes the *Anthrozoös* journal and offers professional meetings and conferences worldwide.

Glossary

acknowledge: to recognize the existence or truth of something.

active listening: to listen for feelings rather than just the factual content of conversations.

attending: body language that lets the person who is talking know that careful attention is being paid to what is being said.

body language: communication through gestures, poses, postures, facial expressions, eye contact, and movements.

clinical communication skills: techniques and strategies necessary for the effective transference of information about diagnosis, prognosis, treatment recommendation, decision making, and end-of-life care.

communicate: to succeed in conveying information; to be connected.

confidentiality: keeping secret or private any information that is entrusted to you about another's personal life.

congruence: an agreement of fit between what is said and what is done.

demonstration: showing or explaining by experience or practical use.

gentle confrontation: using a question or a statement to point out discrepancies or inconsistencies in what has been said or done or used to set limits on clients' behaviors or expectations.

giving permission: encouraging clients to think, feel, and behave however they need to (within safe limits) without fear of judgment.

human-animal bond: a popular way of referring to the types of relationships and attachments people form with animals, particularly companion animals. Also, an accepted area of scholarly research.

immediacy: commenting on what is occurring in the present moment.

nonverbal: a type of communication not involving words or speech.

normalizing: lending credibility to others' thoughts, feelings, behaviors, and experiences.

rapport: a harmonious relationship or communication.

role-play: acting out characters and/or situations as an aid to developing empathy for others as well as improving specific skills and techniques.

self-disclosure: briefly sharing a personal experience when it may be appropriate and of use to someone else.

structuring the environment: adapting the physical elements of an environment to better meet the situation at hand.

support protocol: a written plan of action describing how the various members of the veterinary team can provide guidance, comfort, and follow-up care for clients who are anxious, angry, sad, or grieving.

technique: the skillful use of a tool.

touch: providing comfort and demonstrating care and concern by use of physical contact.

trust: a firm belief in the reliability, truth, or strength of someone or something.

verbal: an oral type of communication; not written.

References

Antelyes, J. "Client Hopes, Client Expectations." *Journal of American Veterinary Medical Association* (1990): 197.

American Veterinary Medical Association. *U.S. Pet Ownership and Demographics Sourcebook.* Schaumburg, IL: AVMA, 2007.

Berlo, D. K. *The Process of Communication: An Introduction to Theory and Practice.* New York: Holt, 1960.

Bristol, D. G. "Using Alumni Research to Assess a Veterinary Curriculum and Alumni Employment and Reward Pattern." *Journal of Veterinary Medical Education* (2002).

Brown, J. P. "The Current and Future Market for Veterinarians and Veterinary Medical Services in the United States." *Journal of American Veterinary Medical Association* (1999): 215.

Coe, J. B., C. L. Adams, and B. N. Bonnett. "A Focus Group Study of Veterinarians and Pet Owners' Perceptions of Veterinarian-Client Communication in Companion Animal Practice." *Journal of American Veterinary Medical Association* 233, no. 7 (2008).

Garland, D. "Workshop Models for Family Life Education: Couples Communication and Negotiation Skills." Family Service Association of America, 1978.

Heath, T. J., and J. N. Mills. "Criteria Used by Employers to Select New Graduate Employees." *Australian Veterinary Journal* (2000).

Holliday, M. *Coaching, Mentoring, and Managing.* Franklin Lakes, New Jersey: Career Press, 2001.

Horvatich, P. K., and K. B. Meyer. "Teaching Client Relations and Communication Skills: Part III—Preliminary Evaluations of Instructional Effectiveness." *Journal of Veterinary Medical Education* (1980).

Kurtz, S. M., T. Laidlaw, G. Makoul et al. "Medical Education Initiatives in Communication Skills." *Cancer Prevention and Control* (1999).

Kurtz, S. M., J. Silverman, and J. Draper. *Teaching and Learning Communication Skills in Medicine.* Abingdon, Oxon, UK: Radcliffe Medical Press, 1998.

Lagoni, L., C. Butler, and S. Hetts. *The Human-Animal Bond and Grief.* Philadelphia, PA: W.B. Saunders, 1994.

Mehrabian, A. "Communication Without Words." *Psychology Today,* September 1968.

Morehead, D., J. Brannan, L. Lagoni, C. Butler, and K. Wheeler. *Guidelines for Bond-Centered Practice.* Fort Collins, CO: Argus Institute, 2001.

The Path to High-Quality Care: Practical Tips for Improving Compliance. Lakewood, CO: AAHA Press, 2003.

Peters, R. *Practical Intelligence.* New York: Harper and Row, 1987.

Schramm, W., ed. "How Communication Works," in *The Process and Effects of Mass Communication.* Urbana: University of Illinois Press, 1954.

Shaw, J. R., B. N. Bonnett, C. L. Adams, and D. L. Roter. "Veterinarian-Client-Patient Communication Patterns Used During Clinical Appointments in Companion Animal Practice." *Journal of American Veterinary Medical Association* 228, no. 5 (2006).

Shaw, J. R., C. L. Adams, and B. N. Bonnett. "What Can Veterinarians Learn from Studies of Physician-Patient Communication About Veterinarian-Client-Patient Communication?" *Journal of American Veterinary Medical Association* 224, no. 5 (2004).

Silverman, J., S. A. Kurtz, and J. Draper. *Skills for Communicating with Patients.* Abingdon, Oxon, UK: Radcliffe Medical Press, 2005.

Stewart, M., J. B. Brown, and W. W. Weston, et al. *Patient-Centered Medicine: Transforming the Clinical Method.* San Francisco: Radcliffe Medical Press, 2003.

Stewart, M. A. "Effective Physician-Patient Communication and Health Outcomes: A Review." *Canadian Medical Association Journal* (1995).

Thompson, D., ed. *The Pocket Oxford Dictionary of Current English,* 8th ed. Oxford: Clarendon Press, 1992.

About the Authors

DANA DURRANCE is a veterinary grief specialist and consultant. She holds two bachelor's degrees from the University of Colorado (one in communication and the other in psychology). She also holds a master's degree in clinical psychology from the University of Colorado and is the former director of the nationally renowned "Changes: Support for People and Pets" program at Colorado State University's James L. Voss Veterinary Teaching Hospital.

Over the past fifteen years, Dana has lectured at more than sixty veterinary conferences, veterinary hospitals, and schools as well as published four books and thirty articles/chapters in veterinary journals and textbooks. She is a regular speaker at Alameda East Veterinary Hospital (home of Animal Planet's *Emergency Vets*). She has also appeared as a grief specialist on ABC's *Good Morning America* and has been featured in the book *The Angel by My Side* (authored by Mike Lingenfelter and David Frei, the spokesman and commentator for USA television and the Westminster Kennel Club).

Dana lives in Colorado Springs, Colorado, with her husband (a veterinarian) and together they own Mountain Shadows Pet Hospital, an AAHA-accredited veterinary hospital. They have a daughter, a son, and three dogs. As both a pet loss counselor and a veterinary practice owner, she has special insight into both pet owners and veterinary professionals.

LAUREL LAGONI is president and CEO of World by the Tail Inc., cocreator and distributor of ClayPaws®, the original paw print kit™, and the director of the Veterinary Wisdom® Resource Center at www.veterinarywisdom.com. Laurel is the cofounder and former director of the Argus Institute for Families and Veterinary Medicine at Colorado State University's James L. Voss Veterinary Teaching Hospital.

Laurel holds a bachelor's degree in journalism from Iowa State University and a master's degree in human development and family studies, with specialties in family therapy and grief education, from Colorado State University. She is the coauthor of four books, including the groundbreaking text *The Human-Animal Bond and Grief* (W.B. Saunders, 1994). Laurel has written more than fifty book chapters and journal articles and has been an invited speaker at numerous national veterinary conferences. She has also lectured at the Smithsonian Institute in Washington, DC. Laurel contributed to *Chicken Soup for the Pet Lover's Soul* and has been showcased on ABC's *20/20* program.

Fort Collins, Colorado, is Laurel's home, where she lives with her husband, two daughters, and several dogs and cats.